T0196069

WHEN GOD DOESN'T HEAL

Avoiding Fear, Shame, and Condemnation

LARRY SILVERMAN

WESTBOW
PRESS®
A DIVISION OF THOMAS NELSON
& ZONDERVAN

Scripture quotations are taken from the Holy Bible, New Living
Translation, copyright ©1996, 2004, 2007, 2013, 2015 by Tyndale
House Foundation. Used by permission of Tyndale House
Publishers, Carol Stream, IL, 60188. All rights reserved.

WestBow Press books may be ordered through booksellers or by contacting:

WestBow Press
A Division of Thomas Nelson & Zondervan
1663 Liberty Drive
Bloomington, IN 47403
www.westbowpress.com
1 (866) 928-1240

Because of the dynamic nature of the Internet, any web addresses or
links contained in this book may have changed since publication and
may no longer be valid. The views expressed in this work are solely those
of the author and do not necessarily reflect the views of the publisher,
and the publisher hereby disclaims any responsibility for them.

Any people depicted in stock imagery provided by Thinkstock are models,
and such images are being used for illustrative purposes only.
Certain stock imagery © Thinkstock.

ISBN: 978-1-9736-0506-5 (sc)
ISBN: 978-1-9736-0507-2 (hc)
ISBN: 978-1-9736-0505-8 (e)

Library of Congress Control Number: 2017914865

Print information available on the last page.

WestBow Press rev. date: 09/28/2017

Endorsements

There's nothing like the testimony and insight of someone who has been there and done that.

This book is the amazing story of a man who has lived for decades in full-time ministry believing in a God who heals, delivers, and always walks with us through the storms of life.

Larry Silverman carefully lays out for us the difference between knowing the truth and walking that truth out; they can be different things.

Throughout this book, you will feel you are going through this entire experience with Larry. Step by step, the author uncovers his emotions from the time his disease was discovered up to the remarkable recovery he is still living out today.

I highly recommend this book to anyone, especially those who are going through a battle with sickness and disease. Questions that arise on this journey include Where is God in all this? Why me? What have I done wrong? Do I lack faith?

Larry does an excellent job dealing with these tough questions and exposing the feelings of condemnation that try to overwhelm us in our times of weakness. This book would make a great gift for anyone facing a health challenge and asking such tough questions.

One of the big revelations for me in reading this book is that Larry brings to light the simple concept that healing is not a matter of faith but of relationship.

This book is a good and easy-to-understand read about a man who has walked through the storm and is still standing!

—Don Keathley
Cofounder and President of Global Grace Seminary and Senior
Pastor of Grace Point Community Church, Houston, TX

In *When God Doesn't Heal: Avoiding Fear, Shame, and Condemnation*, Larry Silverman shares more than a testimony or a story; he lays out his steps toward his healing based on a blueprint of new-covenant grace. He tells of a strong love and marriage filled with faith, healing, and freedom from sickness that is a basic struggle of life. He doesn't write just about his battle with cancer but details the struggles that cancer brings.

My battle was with heart failure accompanied by a heart attack. Your battle may be with depression, a broken relationship, or any number of other problems. In this book, you should find comfort. I found increased faith, strength, and grace on these pages, and so will you. You will not find fear, shame, or condemnation!

—Don Quattlebum
Pastor, River of Life Church, Hugoton, KS

Larry Silverman states, "Many books will suggest ways to be healed and stay healed, but I cannot think of any written about what happens when God doesn't heal."

I highly recommend *When God Doesn't Heal: Avoiding Fear, Shame, and Condemnation* because it goes beyond physical healing though physical healing is important and exactly what Larry desired.

Larry does an outstanding job of establishing the importance of healing from the emotional scars of fear, shame, and condemnation; for many, that is perhaps more important than physical healing. Many who are experiencing deep emotional issues, not only physical issues, can find healing in this open and honest book containing God's truth!

Larry states, "During my cancer journey, I never struggled with fear, shame, or condemnation. I am not suggesting those emotions didn't try to surface, but my resting in God's guidance was strong enough to overcome those emotions when they tried to manifest." Larry recognized his identity in Christ. He said, "I know I am God's son. He didn't give me cancer, nor did cancer enter my life because of my bad lifestyle choices though some of my choices didn't help prevent it either. Yet even there, I chose not to be subjected by fear, shame, or condemnation. It has often been said, "Our attitude is our altitude."

Larry wants you to escape the ultimate killers of fear, shame, and condemnation. Larry said, "These killers are stronger than the sickness and disease itself. My freedom from these emotions was a part of God's mighty healing in my life."

Unfortunately, many people who suffer from negative emotions also suffer from sickness and disease. They are bad enough, but then adding such issues as feeling God is displeased with you makes matters even worse.

The crux of this book is that God loves you; He is not displeased with you. Your current or past condition of sickness and disease has no bearing on His love for you or on your position in Him. Believe God loves you. No matter how sick you are, no matter how great you feel your failure is, Larry wants you to fully experience God's unconditional love for you. He said, "That's where I found my healing, and you as well will find yours there. In 1 John 4:18, we read, "Such love has no fear, because perfect love expels all fear. If we are afraid, it is for fear of punishment, and this shows that we have not fully experienced his perfect love."

—Dr. Cecil Cockerham
Cofounder and Vice President of Global Grace Seminary

CONTENTS

Dedication

As I did with my first book, I dedicate this book to the best wife in the world and to three other groups of people.

No words can describe how wonderful my wife was and continues to be as we walk out my battle with cancer. During my long hospital stay, Corinne would drive ninety minutes each way often through heavy rain on one of the most accident-prone stretches of expressway in the country—Interstate 75. Prior to my illness, there would be no way she would every drive on an expressway! My doctors and nurses were extremely impressed with the dedication, love, and support she showed me. I remember the times right before I went to sleep that she called me and prayed with me even though I couldn't talk. What comfort! Corinne led my guardian angel team. What a gal!

Along with my wife, I dedicate this book to my great family, especially my children. One of the positive side effects of my cancer battle is the wonderful healing and uniting effect it had on my family. Many of my family members gathered in the surgical waiting room at Shands Hospital for the twelve-hour wait. The hospital staff was greatly impressed, and great family support continues.

Third, I dedicate this book to all my caregivers, my guardian angels. They include many doctors, nurses, hospital staff members, home health care support, and a larger group of people way too many to mention by name. I am alive today because God chose this huge group of caregivers. There is no way I can state how much these people mean to me.

Last, I dedicate this book to the greatest church group in the world, all the members of New Covenant Grace Fellowship in Inverness, Florida. These people continued to pray for both of us, but they went way beyond the call of duty. We never had to rely on outside, substitute ministry. These people carried the load and did an outstanding job doing so. Thanks so much to all who attend the neatest church in Florida!

Foreword

Salvage Procedure

It was early morning. I had gotten to work early to have some quiet time to go through referrals and test reports before my patients came in. This had been my practice since I started my career as a physician's assistant over thirty years previously.

I read the words again and tried to look beyond them. I had been in this office for over ten years, and many of my patients had become family. They shared their children's and grandchildren's trials and successes with me each time they came in. Each heart attack, each case of pneumonia, each cancer diagnosis struck a little more personally because of these relationships. But I had been in the "business" long enough to have heard these words a few times and to understand what "salvage procedure" implied. Those two words spoke volumes to me—prolonged surgeries with numerous specialty surgeons crowded around a body each waiting to step up to the table and add their expertise to a huge medical procedure that would mean months if not years of struggle and compromise and of learning innovative ways of doing the mundane—swallowing, breathing, speaking—that list was endless.

It was then that I saw it; the name of the poor soul who would find himself on that OR table: "Silverman, Larry."

Larry and his wife, Corinne, had begun coming to the office a few years earlier. They were both reasonably healthy, so aside from routine visits, I heard little from them. Unfortunately, Larry had recently been diagnosed with cancer of the mouth. That resulted in my having to slog through endless paperwork and deal with his insurance company. He had undergone a simple dental extraction several months earlier. Because the wound did not heal properly, a biopsy was performed. Since then, Larry needed to have all his teeth adjacent to the original tooth removed, but no oral surgeon in our area was willing to deal with a biopsy-proven malignancy. He had been referred to an oral surgeon who had advised that he be seen by maxillofacial surgeon, who had advised that he see an oncologist, who had advised that he start by having the teeth removed by of all people a dentist.

Finally, he had been referred to the University of Florida's Shands Hospital's ear, nose, and throat department, the mecca for all the big stuff that required a higher level of medical expertise than the norm. The last I had heard, Larry's insurance had refused the requested referral. However surprisingly now, I held the letter from Shands, and the words *salvage procedure* were in the first two sentences. Larry and his wife would be in that morning, and we'd have to discuss this.

I shook my head. All I could think of was the enormity of the procedure and whether someone, anyone, had taken the time to give them details about what awaited them. I've always believed that post-op "surprises" are unacceptable and that every person deserves all the information available before the day of surgery. There are always things that occur during surgery that require some changes in plans because of unforeseen problems.

However, a salvage procedure is different. It's the kind of surgery that most surgeons only read about and that no patient wants to experience.

The morning began. I knocked on the exam room door and stepped through the doorway praying for the right words and to be calm enough to address their anxieties and answer at least some of their questions. It had been many years since I had been a part of this kind of situation, and I knew I'd not be able to give them many details as ear, nose, and throat oncology was not part of my background.

As I met Larry's eyes, I was taken aback. All I saw in his and his wife's eyes was peace. I smiled and started to gently sift through what information they had been given and how much they understood about what the next few weeks would mean to them.

The visit went well. Larry told me everything they knew about the upcoming procedure. His voice was strong, and he held my gaze throughout our visit. He explained the planned bone transplant that would replace the portion of his jawbone that needed to be removed due to the tumor. He informed me about the plan for a feeding tube as the mouth and throat tissue healed and slowly returned to the jobs they had been made for.

Corinne sat quietly at his side listening and holding his hand. She said nothing but let him own this time and the explanation of the fight he was embarking on. She silently stated her support for her spouse of so many years.

When he finished, I tried to set the stage for them by telling them that this would be a very big deal and that they had a long road ahead of them. No matter what I said, all I saw was peace resting on both. This led me to think, *They have no idea what's coming their way.*

Unfortunately, I recalled Mr. T, whose liver was rapidly failing. He was suffering with end-stage kidney failure, dementia, diabetes, and coronary artery disease, and he had been placed on a transplant list. At seventy-five, his health was poor. He and his wife were convinced to agree to this enormous procedure, and he went to surgery.

Two weeks after receiving his new liver and after a myriad of tests including cardiac catheterization and having to start dialysis while he was still in the ICU, he passed away. I was not there when he and Janet, his wife of many years, spoke to the transplant team. Yet even now, I marvel that anyone would even consider a procedure of this magnitude for this man. The adage "Dum spiro, spero" (While I breathe, I hope) is true. It often seems that modern medicine does some things simply because they can be done instead of helping patients prepare for the next stage of life, which often involves death.

I spent the rest of the day wondering if I were off the mark in my thinking about the same possible outcome for Larry. I prayed for the surgeons, the people Larry and Corinne had spoken to and made plans with.

Then the countdown began. Larry had given me the scheduled date for his surgery, and I spent at least a part of each day praying for his safety and healing and peace for him and his wife.

I've had a personal relationship with Jesus Christ since my teens. I had seen my prayers answered too many times not to know Larry could awake one morning cancer-free. I'd seen broken marriages healed overnight because God had heard the prayers of one small person. I'd read the accounts of the blind man and the leper Jesus healed. I knew there were at least two other people in my office who were lifting this man up in prayer.

Our entire office then waited.

It was several more weeks before Larry returned to the office. I never check my daily schedule because too often I'd prepared for a visit only to have a patient cancel at the last minute or not show up at all. Each day, I deal with who comes in instead of preparing for the what ifs.

When Larry and Corinne came in, I had only a few minutes to read the surgery notes before I stepped into the exam room. Larry was seated next to his wife. There it was again—complete peace. He was significantly thinner than when I'd seen him last, but the anxiety and frustration of this huge ordeal was not there. Corinne, his tiny wife, whom I had never perceived as a strong person, glowed with peace. They told me about Larry's twelve-hour procedure that had gone off without a hitch. He spoke of having no pain and about being fussed at by his nurses for not using his on-demand pain med pump. He told me for the first time about their walk with the Lord and how he had gone into the operating room that day with complete peace. They shared about their prayers for healing and what they were learning through this challenging time.

I saw Larry and Corinne sporadically during the following weeks. However, the surgeons kept me up-to-date with notes from each visit. Not long after Larry went home, he developed a fistula under his chin; that's an abnormal connection between two spaces that can occur during surgery or can come about, as in his case, by significant inflammation possibly due to radiation treatments. Larry had developed an infection with lots of drainage from this opening. They made the ninety-minute trip to Shands again and were seen that morning by their surgeon. This opening was enlarged to allow drainage and then packed with a sterile dressing to keep the wound open and draining.

Because of where the fistula was, it required twice-daily packing changes as it drained and healed slowly. The ninety-minute trip each way would be more than daunting because Larry was still very weak from everything he had been through.

Enter Nurse Corinne. For the next several weeks, she cleaned this wound and repacked it with a cool confidence that I would never have expected of her. She seemed oblivious to the nasty drainage, the open wound, and the process of placing numerous inches of sterile dressing tightly in a seemingly small wound.

It's been several months since Larry's surgery. His wounds have healed, and he is feeling terrific. His speech is not the same as it was, and I don't expect it ever will be. He has some issues with food particles and saliva getting lost in portions of his mouth and throat, which aren't working as they should. He has continued to lose weight, but that's something he does by choice. He can eat just about anything, and the feeding tube is now only a small scar and a memory.

I have seen many people go through what I see as Hades on earth with medical issues. Surgeries of this magnitude often leave patients frail and stressed for months. The outcome is often less than perfect. The frustrations of reworking daily activities often lead people to deep despair. There are so many accounts of patients who relive significant life stresses after having been under anesthesia. That frequently results in deep clinical depression with implications of its own. But Larry had very little of that.

More and more, I hear of surgeons who pray with their patients and the OR staff before surgeries. What a comfort to know that the big guys—the doctors and nurses who stand with their patients during the challenging times—understand that God alone is the Healer who has our lives in His precious right hand every second.

But Larry's story is far from complete. I have cared for patients who, when faced with significant illness, have turned to their Christian friends and family for help and support only to be told they had not been healed because they hadn't prayed enough, because they had sin in their lives, or because they didn't have enough faith. I always tell these people that their friends and family need to come to know the true God, the sovereign One who knows the ending before we even know there is a beginning. His ways are far above ours, and His plan always ends the same way—in healing one way or another. Larry's plan was to help tell this story.

My pastor of many years, a truly godly man, lost his only child to a malignant brain tumor when the boy was not quite sixteen. He has struggled, wept, and struggled again. I marveled as this man talked the talk and walked the walk. Through his son's illness and since his death, he always spoke with power and conviction even when his heart was shattered and he felt he could not take another breath. God had shown him that *healing* has many meanings. I pray you will see this truth in Larry's inspired and heartfelt book.

I thank Pastors Larry and Corinne Silverman for letting me be a tiny part of their incredible journey. I have grown because of them and by their witness to a truth far greater than that of modern medicine.

—Gretchen Kronenthal, PA-C (Larry's Primary Care)

INTRODUCTION

My cell phone rang around 11:00 a.m. on January 2, 2016. It was the receptionist from the oral surgeon's office, where a biopsy sample of my mouth had been taken on Christmas Eve. Her message to me was very emphatic. "The doctor wants to see you right away, today."

I asked, "Is it cancer?"

She replied, "The doctor will fill you in when you get here."

With a lump in my throat, I informed Corinne. We ate a quick lunch and headed to Ocala, about thirty minutes north.

The doctor informed us that I had a form of skin cancer, squamous cell carcinoma, in my gum line on the lower left side. His voice was gentle and calm as he told us of some of the options we had, but his first suggestion was for us to contact the University of Florida's ear, nose, and throat department for a consultation on the possibilities of surgery. That option soon led to a frustrating dead end, one that possibly could have caused my death and did lead to several complications due to my insurance company—complications I'm still dealing with.

The following Sunday immediately after the service, I gathered the leaders of our church and filled them in on the details. The next Sunday, I announced my situation to our church. They were stunned, but they immediately began praying for me; many laid hands on me as tears streamed down their faces. I wanted to go public with my situation; I had nothing to hide. I began a Facebook page, Update on Larry, so I could keep family and friends informed. Several hundred Facebook friends asked to join the page, all offering lots of prayer and support. I was prayed for by many pastors and ministers from all over the country, many whom we knew as we had ministered in their churches.

Though we felt we wanted to proceed with the direction my doctors suggested, we never lost sight of the fact that God was my healer. I fully expected the tumor to shrink and disappear. I also felt I would soon spit the tumor out.

For many years, I prayed and declared usually several times per week, "No cancer can ever live in my body. If there is any cancer present, it must die and harmlessly pass from my body." It was because I felt I was doing everything right. I had prayed for many people and had witnessed God heal them. I saw many instant miracles as well as slow healings take place in the lives of others over my many years of ministry. Therefore, I knew I was a strong candidate for a miracle myself as my faith in God's healing power was operating near 100 percent.

Yet I wasn't healed. At least not in the way I would have chosen. Nevertheless, God was strongly at work in me and through the ministrations of others to bring a far greater healing in my body and ultimately my life.

This is my story, one I trust will encourage you and help you understand God's working in your life. Through my walk through my valley of the shadow of death, I avoided the pitfalls of destruction that fear, shame, and condemnation can cause. I want to help you avoid these traps as well.

If you're dealing with a health issue and feel you haven't been healed by God, I have good news for you in this book. After all, He is the Lord who heals us!

1

More Background

Millions of Christians have given their testimonies, written books, and produced videos about God's miraculous healing power in their lives. Often through prayer and the laying on of hands, their illnesses were dramatically healed.

However, multitudes of sick people, folks who are in love with God and have sought Him for their healing, remain sick or even die. These people have not shared healing testimonies, written books, or produced videos about their experiences. Instead, they often feel God had deserted them, and as a result, they live their remaining days in fear, shame, and condemnation.

I am very thankful for those who have been healed, but I have a passion for those who have had their healing escape them. Recently, I unexpectedly found myself part of that latter group. But through my intense experiences, I discovered some interesting truths about God and especially about myself.

I believe in the healing power of God. I have witnessed too many miracles in myself, my wife, and many others to deny God still heals the sick. I believe that it is His will to heal and that no sickness and disease comes from God to teach someone a lesson.

For many years, my wife and I traveled the country preaching and practicing Hebrews 13:8: "Jesus Christ is the same yesterday, today and forever." We have personally witnessed many, many people freed from sickness and disease, so I can never deny what God has done and continues to do so often for those who seek Him in healing.

But for as many people as I have seen healed, I have seen many who have not been healed. It is to that group of dedicated warriors that I wish to minister through this book. I trust that my story of my journey will bless and encourage them.

In late September 2015, I noticed that a molar in my lower jaw seemed to be getting loose. Initially, I didn't think too much about it because both my molars in that area had been removed due to root canals going bad. I thought I was dealing with just another bad tooth.

But over the next several weeks, the tooth loosened more, so I visited my dentist in late November. She felt it was best to remove the tooth. I was looking at a partial plate to fill in for the removed molars anyway. The tooth was extracted, and my mouth seemed to heal properly.

However, a couple of weeks later, I noticed that the swelling and discomfort around the extraction site were increasing. I revisited my dentist, who said, "I suspected a problem when I extracted that tooth and suggest that you have a biopsy performed."

On Christmas Eve 2015, an oral surgeon took a biopsy of my gum area and sent it to the University of Florida's lab in Gainesville.

The day after New Year's Day 2016, the oral surgeon's office called and told me that the doctor wanted to see me right away. My wife, Corinne, and I immediately drove to the surgeon in Ocala. The biopsy report showed a case of squamous cell carcinoma, a normally slow-growing type of skin cancer.

Of course, our little world was quickly shaken. The dreaded *C* word had been pronounced upon my life. The oral surgeon quickly assured us that this type of cancer was very treatable and that due to its growing outward instead of inward, the treatment outcome would be very favorable. He suggested I seek treatment at the University of

Florida Shands Hospital's ear, nose, and throat department as the people there had a lot of experience in this area.

However, insurance problems soon arose, and I was not authorized for this treatment. Instead, my primary doctor in my HMO network referred me to an oncologist for chemo and radiation treatments. But prior to any radiation treatments, I'd have to have all my lower teeth extracted. That created another problem—my insurance wouldn't authorize any oral surgeons in my network who could deal with the cancer issues.

I had many rounds of strong chemotherapy without radiation. The tumor shrunk with each round of chemo, but it soon grew back larger than before. After many weeks of patiently waiting with chemo treatments only and visiting several oral surgeons who refused to pull my teeth because of the cancer, I was finally authorized to have my teeth extracted by UF's oral surgery department.

Daily radiation treatments began within a few weeks and lasted for seven weeks. I also had more weekly chemo treatments. The tumor was greatly reduced but never eradicated.

After the radiation ended, I had several weeks' rest. During that time, the tumor seemed to grow, and the discomfort was unbearable. I also had many mouth sores, a side effect of the chemo and radiation. Because of the side effects and loss of my lower teeth, eating became very selective and difficult. I needed to lose weight, but that was not the way to accomplish it.

The results of a CT scan were very negative. The cancer had spread to the lymph nodes in my neck. My radiation oncologist was very concerned and made waves with my insurance company. I was finally authorized to see an ear, nose, and throat surgeon at the University of Florida Shands Hospital in Gainesville. That was where I had wanted to go months earlier but had been denied.

There, I was told I'd need salvage surgery. The surgeon told me I had a 40 percent chance of being cancer-free post-surgery. Corinne and I were stunned when we learned the plan of treatment. I'd need an immediate G tube inserted in my stomach so I could have just liquid food after the operation, which would take twelve hours and require three surgeons to work on me simultaneously.

Most of my lower jawbone would be removed because the cancer had also penetrated it. The smaller bone from my right leg, my fibula, would be removed and made into a new jawbone. Some of my mouth and tongue would also be removed as the cancer had spread there as well. A section of flesh from my right leg would be removed and attached in my mouth to form a flap. My neck would be sliced from end to end below my jaw so all the lymph nodes could be removed. I'd have to endure a tracheotomy so I could breathe properly. I would be hospitalized for three weeks followed by a week or so of rehab. Corinne and I were in shock.

I underwent a full twelve hours of surgery on Thursday, September 15, 2016, but the outcome was very good—all signs of cancer were removed. Later, pathology reports came back that all the cancer had been eliminated. I am now awaiting five years of no more cancer signs so I can be officially declared cancer-free.

Prior to this long, drawn-out ordeal, I had received much prayer. My church, New Covenant Grace Fellowship in Inverness, Florida, prayed intensively over me. I received prayer from an evangelist noted for many miracle healings in his ministry as well as from family and many friends. Five thousand Facebook friends continued to hold me up in prayer. I had received all this prayer and had sought God for healing and deliverance, but I wasn't healed.

Or was I? That's the rest of my story.

2

FEAR, SHAME, AND CONDEMNATION

Fear, shame, and condemnation are three of the greatest enemies a Christian can face. The three-work hand in hand to destroy those who believe in Jesus Christ. Unfortunately, we witness far too much of their influence in the church today.

Over the past several years, the Holy Spirit opened my eyes to the biblical truths of new- covenant grace. Understanding this new way of life radically transformed my life and those of my family and church. No longer do we strive to live under a list of laws thinking that by doing so we will be more pleasing in God's sight and thus receive more answers to our prayers.

One of the discoveries of this new life has been that law—any law, not just the law of Moses in the old covenant—will always end up leading a person to fear, shame, and condemnation because God did not design us to be able to completely follow law. Instead, we live under a new law of love that enters our lives through faith in the finished works of Christ on His cross.

I went into full-time ministry in 1976. Throughout many of those years, I lived by and taught a mixed message of law and grace. One of the greatest lies I ever taught went something like this: The more we please God, the more He will be pleased with us and answer our prayers. The newfound truth that grace afforded to that lie is that God, through Christ, is already pleased with us and that we to simply to rest in His wonderful grace.

When I began to understand God's marvelous plan for my life, I realized that others had taught me most of what I had been teaching; I was a product of my teachers. There's nothing wrong with being a product of your teachers if what your teachers taught you was correct. However, I find that much of what is taught in today's church is incorrect; it often results from misinterpreting scripture and adhering to tradition. As I began to see this in myself, I was appalled.

I realized that much of my teaching was legalistic; I was setting up laws for myself and others to follow. The result was setting up myself and others for failure. We could not live up to what I was teaching, and we were left with fear, shame, and condemnation.

During the early days of my Christian experience, Corinne and I attended a medium-sized but rapidly growing Pentecostal church. I later became associate pastor of that church. The pastor taught a strong healing and deliverance message; as a result, many were healed and delivered from sickness and disease. The pastor was regionally known as a faith healer. Many would visit our church and often receive the miracles they sought. But unfortunately, many left services not having been healed. However, we didn't hear too much from them. Healing and deliverance became a type of law in that church. I can explain this by a personal event.

Prior to my faith in Christ, I was plagued by constant, bad headaches brought on by business stress. The back of my neck was always tight, and tension radiated up my neck into my head causing tremendous pain by the end of the day. It seemed that by living in my newfound faith in Christ, the tightness was eliminated and the headaches pretty much ceased.

Then one Sunday morning at church, an immense "pounder" hit my head. I prayed, but the headache remained. That seemed strange; prior to that, I'd pray and the headache would immediately cease.

On the way home from the service, I told Corinne I wanted to pick up some pain medication; we had tossed out all pain medication in our home as an act of faith. I hadn't needed any in months.

To make matters worse, the implication that I had from the church's teaching was that to have to resort to painkillers was a lack of faith on my part. That concept was not directly taught, but the implication was solidly there.

By that time, I was in a leadership position in the church and didn't want any witnesses to my lack of faith. I snuck into the store, picked up the medication, and slunk to the checkout lanes. I felt like a spy on a secret mission. Thankfully, the store was not very busy, so the chances of my stealth run for pain relief would most likely go unnoticed and my reputation as a man of faith would remain intact.

But as I set the bottle of pain medication in front of the cashier, I heard a familiar voice: "Brother Larry! What are you doing here?" It was Brother Howard, whom I had sat close to in church an hour earlier. Busted! Howard said he was there for a birthday cake for his wife. I stood there with the evidence of my lack of faith sitting in front of that cashier. I felt embarrassed and condemned.

You must think this story is absurd, but it really happened. I was trying to follow the implied law of our church regarding healing and medication. I felt I had failed God because I needed pain medication. I was demonstrating all three—fear, shame, and condemnation. I was fearful that someone might discover my lack of faith, and when that happened, I felt shame that led to condemnation. I felt guilty for not having enough faith to get healed from a headache. I thought I must not have been a good Christian.

Here is what I realized. Many in the body of Christ today have made healing a type of law. Many believe the reason God hasn't healed them is because they don't have enough faith to be healed. I am sorry to report such concepts have indeed been taught in the American church and have spread worldwide.

In the early days of my battle with cancer, Corinne and I decided to act in one accord. We sought God together about what our course of action should be. One choice was that we could battle this thing solely through our faith in God. We also saw we could combine our faith with very rigid nutritional treatment. Or we could follow the designs of the medical community. We decided to follow medical advice; we believed God would lead my doctors as we sought divine healing and deliverance.

Right from the start, we gently told people to mind their own business as we had witnessed way too many cancer patients being bombarded by others declaring a need to eat certain foods and quote certain Bible verses. Our thought was that if God wanted us to go down any of those avenues, He would show us and we would know for certain if people's advice was warranted.

One faith teacher suggested to me that a cancer sufferer to whom he had ministered daily walked around his property quoting healing verses of scripture and that I should do likewise. He later told others in our church that people (me) were sick in our church because we didn't preach healing every week! Can you see the formation of law here? I have often wondered how in the world those living in the days of the early church had made it without Bibles to read and quote. Yet the saints of the early church endured and overcame persecution that would make a modern American church attendee wilt with fear.

Many books will suggest ways to be healed and stay healed, but I cannot think of any written about what happens when God doesn't heal. Because of our modern means of communication including books, social media, and television, modern Christians have information and knowledge piled on them. Paul told Timothy that in the last days, people would "be always learning but never able to come to a knowledge of the truth" (2 Timothy 3:7). It appears that we are living in those times. Learning that leads to knowledge is a good thing, but if it is based on untruths, only damaging results can follow.

During my cancer journey, I never struggled with fear, shame, or condemnation. I am not suggesting those emotions didn't try to surface, but my resting in God's guidance was strong enough to overcome those emotions when they tried to manifest. I know I am

God's son. He didn't give me cancer, nor did cancer enter my life because of my bad lifestyle choices though some of my choices didn't help prevent it either. Yet even there, I chose not to be subjected by fear, shame, or condemnation.

With this book, I trust I can help you also escape the ultimate killers: fear, shame, and condemnation, which are stronger than sickness and disease. My freedom from those emotions was a part of God's mighty healing in my life.

There is no way to fully comprehend just how damaging fear, shame, and condemnation can be to humanity let alone just those who call themselves Christians. But based on my years of pastoral duties and counseling experience, I know that many Christians, maybe even most, are plagued by these emotions in one form or another. It saddens me to think that many of those who suffer these horrible emotions also suffer from sickness and disease at the same time. Let's face it—sickness and disease are bad enough, but to add such issues as feeling God is displeased with them and is punishing them because of their lack of faith makes matters that much worse.

God loves you and is not displeased with you. Your current or past condition of sickness and disease has no bearing on His love for you and on your position in Him. It's imperative that you believe that.

In Ephesians, Paul prayed over the people he has ministered to in Ephesus. In our church, we discovered that these Ephesian prayers were interesting and relevant to our new-covenant walk with Christ. In Ephesians 3:18–20, Paul prayed,

> And may you have the power to understand, as all God's people should, how wide, how long, how high, and how deep his love is. May you experience the love of Christ, though it is too great to understand fully. Then you will be made complete with all the fullness of life and power that comes from God.

9

Larry Silverman

I agree with Paul in his prayers for the Ephesian church and include you in them as well. I too ask God to show you just how great His love for you really is though you will never fully understand it. No matter how sick you are, no matter how much you feel you have failed God, I want you to experience His full love. That's where I found my healing, and you as well will find yours there.

3

WHY DOESN'T EVERYONE GET HEALED?

(This chapter is an introduction to the next several chapters)

For many years, I have written a blog, "The River Is Here" (larrysilverman.blogs.com). Based on this blog, a few years ago, I wrote my first book, *The River Is Here: My Journey into New Covenant Grace.* I based it on my blog posts of my journey into the revelations of new-covenant grace. My format in the book was to copy a past blog post into a new chapter. After the blog post, I would include additional comments.

During the dark days of cancer, I couldn't write as many posts as I would have desired to. Many days, especially for a couple of months prior to surgery, I spent a lot of time in bed as I didn't have enough energy to do anything. However, I did manage to write a few new posts both pre- and post-surgery. Therefore, I would like to include these posts in the next few chapters as I feel my message is relevant especially as these posts reflect my feelings during those days of darkness.

In these chapters, I will use the same format as my prior book—a blog post and follow-up comments. Due to the nature of the blogs, there will be some repetition involved, but please bear with me as any repetitive thoughts should be beneficial.

Blog Post: June 18, 2016

I have waited a long time to write this and the next post. I've done a lot of soul searching, praying, meditating, and reading my Bible to investigate this subject more fully. So, this isn't some knee-jerk reaction to things going on in my body

I believe in the healing properties of God without a doubt. I embrace this belief as I've seen way too much to not believe in it. In all my years of ministry, I have prayed for (ministered to) maybe hundreds of people who have been healed as I laid hands on them. Even members of my family have been healed, including my wife and children.

I remember the day the doctor told my wife she had cancer. Later, it was gone; the Lord had done the healing! It didn't come from medical treatment but from the ministry of the Holy Spirit.

I've been healed of many things over the years as well—from bad head colds to severe back problems and some issues worse that those. So yes, I am a believer in the healing power of God.

When I was told this past January that I had stage-3 cancer in my mouth, my little world was traumatized but my faith in God's healing power wasn't the least bit shaken. I expected a miracle at any moment. Corinne and I had complete peace about seeking medical treatment. I recall in days gone by that I made rash statements such as, "If I ever have cancer, I'll *never* submit to chemotherapy or radiation!" But we felt total peace in seeking medical help, which included chemo and radiation, yet all the time, we expected the healing from God to manifest.

I have learned a very important lesson about healing issues—no one has all the answers on the subject. Some preachers seem to know it all, but they don't. One famous "faith preacher" would chastise those in his congregation if they ever went to a doctor, but he had to wear a lift in one shoe because one leg was shorter than the other. Another wore a micro hearing aid so people he ministered to didn't know he had hearing issues.

If you ever run across people who tell you they have all the answers on healing, run for your life; they're lying. I'm not ashamed to tell you I don't have all the answers on this subject, but I'll keep ministering healing no matter what. What happens after that is up to God.

From the onset of my condition, I made it clear I didn't want to hear all the formulas, diets, lifestyle changes, etc., that some well-meaning folks wanted to see me embrace. Corinne and I felt certain we had a clear-cut path to walk, and that was what we did.

Still, one guy suggested that every message in our church had to proclaim healing. I was also told I needed to confess more of the Word. It was even suggested that I should walk around our property declaring healing scriptures daily. It seems that when it comes to cancer, everyone has a pet cure.

Having evaluated these things, we quickly ascertained that most of them came from works, thus forming a law. How much scripture must I confess daily before God destroys the cancer in my mouth? When do I declare the Word enough for the healing to be manifested? How many healing messages do I need to hear in our church for God's healing to manifest? For Corinne and me, the answer was zero. All that stuff is works—law—and leads only to condemnation. Yes, condemnation. If I don't do enough for healing to take place, that means there's something wrong with me. Condemnation is the only thing that can follow that thinking.

Have people been healed by walking around their property confessing healing scriptures? I'm sure some have been. Yet is that God's method for everyone? If you think so, I have a bridge to sell you.

I'll write more on this subject in the days to come; my heart is very full. If you're dealing with condemnation in your own journey to health, if you're wondering what more you can do for God to heal you, you're on the path of condemnation that leads nowhere. Instead, please rest in the finished works of Jesus Christ, think about what he has done for you, and watch what He will do for you.

About my condition ... Monday, I finish the last dose of

radiation, over seven weeks of it. I will also complete the weekly chemo treatments. The tumor has dramatically been reduced, but it is not totally gone. The radiation is to keep on working for a month or so, so I'll be waiting on what the future holds. In the meantime, I still give all the glory to God for my healing. I am quick to say, "I've been healed by the stripes of Jesus Christ."

I also refuse to live under the veil of condemnation; I'm too good for that because Jesus has made me righteous and holy.

More on this subject later—grace and peace!

Additional Comments

How I remember what my life was like during the days when I wrote the above blog. I wasn't really discouraged, but I was frustrated—not with God but with insurance companies.

I have mentioned previously that I needed all my lower teeth extracted because the radiation would weaken my jawbone and any dental work could possibly do great damage or even break my jaw.

At the time, I had no idea that I would eventually have most of my lower jaw removed and replaced by a very intense surgical procedure. The insurance company I was dealing with was an HMO. They thought it necessary for the sake of their profit margin to make certain I had my teeth extracted by an in-network oral surgeon. The problem was that none in our area would pull my teeth because of the cancer.

We fought the insurance company for many weeks until we decided we could no longer afford to wait for the insurance to pay. We decided to self-pay the oral surgery department at the University of Florida. Just a few minutes before the teeth were to be pulled, the insurance company called to say it would cover the procedure, and we got our check back. That was great, but the long wait of several weeks had been very damaging—the cancer had become more entrenched in my mouth.

My level of frustration increased greatly. However, even amid great frustration, I found inner peace. Somedays, I had to look deep to find it, but I always did. I don't know what I would have done without it. And Corinne had it too. I'm certain her battles were different from mine as she continuously saw me getting weaker every day.

My mouth sores were bad those days. Both chemo and radiation were making it very difficult for me to eat. Some days, even drinking water was a chore. I could eat chicken noodle soup and very bland foods. Eventually, salty foods, including the soup, would hurt, and so did sugar of any kind. I tried to avoid a lot of sugar because it possibly fed cancer. What we didn't know at the time was that the chemo and radiation didn't completely eradicate the tumor and that the cancer was beginning to spread into lymph nodes in my neck on the right side; the nodes on the left side had already been destroyed by the radiation treatments. Cancer was also beginning to spread in my mouth and tongue. These spots were very irritated by the cancer and caused me more eating difficulties.

I have ministered to numerous cancer patients, many with huge tumors in other parts of their bodies. I had observed people deal with very severe pain as a result. Here I was dealing with such a small tumor at least compared to others, but this thing was physically eating my lunch.

I could have wondered why I wasn't getting healed by God; I could have been asking, "God, why me?" I could have done a spiritual checkup to find out what I was doing wrong and thus hindering God from healing me. Even with medical help, my situation was getting worse. Not only was God not healing me; it seemed that the doctors weren't either. What a mess!

Yet deep within me was God's peace, a special gift. I believe that gift of peace is in all who face sickness and disease. I'm certain you have the same gift of peace in you. Even if you feel God hasn't healed you, that gift of peace continues to dwell within. Please take some time today and look in yourself. Remember that Jesus' last words were, "It is finished." That means you don't have to wait for Him to heal you because He already has.

However, the rub comes when you do not see and maybe never see the healing manifested. We will consider this more later in this book. However, in the meantime, I suggest that God always heals the sick; it just doesn't always come the way we think it should. Yes, even death can be a form of God's healing. We'll look at that later also.

As for now, let it suffice to say, "So now there is no condemnation for those who belong to Christ Jesus" (Romans 8:1) That is you, my friend. Though you may be sick or near death, fear, shame, and condemnation do not belong to you, so never claim them.

4

Why Doesn't Everyone Get Healed? Part 2

Blog Post: June 25, 2016

To fully understand this post, scroll down and read the first in the series [the previous chapter]. That way, you'll read this in context.

The title is, "Why Doesn't Everyone Get Healed?" This title is a little confusing because I believe everyone does get healed no matter what the symptoms look like on any one day. Even in death, there's healing. I know some do not understand that, but to a believer in Christ, death is no longer an enemy. So, if you are indeed a believer, you can never be defeated by health issues.

As I stated in the first post, when I learned I had cancer in my mouth, my little world came to a halt. The first thing I had to face was that my life for some time to come would look very different from what it had looked like prior to the prognosis. I certainly determined that correctly.

Wow! How things have changed. Everything in my life is different now than it was even six months ago. Some things will never return to the normal of those days. For instance, I had to have all my lower teeth pulled prior to radiation because after radiation, I wouldn't be allowed to have any major dental work done for two years. It's not a good thing for a person like me, who enjoys tasty food, to be relegated to not eating it. For instance, I had a grilled cheese sandwich last night for supper, but I had to cut it up and soak it in soup to eat it. See what I mean? If you're going through any major health issues, be prepared for a changed life.

Regardless, I believe God has healed me. Though I still have some of the tumor, I'm convinced I was healed two thousand years ago. I have no idea why I'm still dealing with symptoms, but they don't diminish my faith in Christ's working in me one bit.

I have many people praying for me, and I so appreciate that. However, I was very careful especially in the early days when it came to asking for prayer. What I didn't want was a bunch of clever ideas on how to get rid of cancer. Here is a fact—I *can* hear from God. And you can too.

When Job's comforters show up telling you that you must have secret sin in your life, or that you're not quoting enough "healing" verses, or that you just don't have enough faith—on and on—just turn your face from that nonsense. Trust that if you have a problem in one of those areas, God will make it plain to you.

Healing is not a big mystery. You don't have to do everything just right to be healed. If you're going down a road like that, you're on the wrong road. The new covenant is one of rest and peace. If you're experiencing anything other than rest and peace, if you're under condemnation, you're on the wrong road.

A few years ago, Bruce, a dear brother in our church, was diagnosed with a very vicious form of cancer. It seemed that just a couple of weeks after the cancer was made known, he began going downhill fast. Our church ministered to him in every way we knew how. We prayed and laid hands on him many times. We counseled him the best we could, but Bruce became frailer daily. In a few weeks, he was bedridden.

Corrine and I and several other families brought food in for him and his wife. Once when we came with a meal, I could tell Bruce was very troubled. He felt condemned by the fact he wasn't healed. I felt the Lord wanted me to tell him he was okay. I told him it was even okay for him to die. As I encouraged Bruce, I saw the condemnation breaking off him.

A few days later, Bruce passed away. He did so in the perfect will of God. He had total peace. It was time for Bruce to go home and remain for eternity in God's presence. Who can say Bruce wasn't perfectly healed?

Here's some good advice—stay away from Job's comforters. They are religious people who will lead you only into condemnation. Listen to the Holy Spirit within you. If He wants you to eat different food, He'll tell you. If He wants you to quote healing verses, He'll tell you. If He wants you to see Doctor X instead of Doctor Y, He'll tell you. Then rest, my friend. God is overseeing your destiny.

Here's how I'm handling this cancer affliction. I'm living and overcoming one day at a time. I'm following my doctors' advice, but I'm doing that with one eye on Jesus because I know that any day, the miracle of total healing will take place. I expect to one day spit the remaining tumor out. If it comes any other way, well, I'm okay with that too. I just know I was healed, and I know you were too. Glory be to God.

Grace and peace!

Additional Comments

It is very thought provoking for me to read these two old blog posts; what memories they bring back. So much has changed in my life since I wrote them, which seems decades ago.

Today is April 15, 2017, the day before Easter. Resurrection has much greater meaning to me this year. It's 10:35 a.m. Exactly seven months ago, I was in the operating room at Shands Hospital undergoing a twelve-hour surgical procedure, one that saved my life. I didn't know then that chemo and radiation therapy would change my life so radically.

In the blog posts, I wrote of my extreme belief in God's healing supremacy for me. I mentioned a couple of times that I felt that any time I would spit the cancer out, but Corrine and I were convinced it was so important for me to go through the medical treatment my doctors had suggested. Our faith in God's healing provision for me never wavered, but the miracle we were expecting never materialized. That salvage surgery was the only option left, but even then, I was expecting a miracle.

Corinne and I often recall the words of Dr. Brian Boyce, my ear, nose, and throat doctor and surgeon. We'll never forget the shock we felt when he told us about what my surgical procedure would require. I sat in the examining chair listening to him but feeling completely numb to his words; I couldn't believe he was talking to me. I had a minor cancer in my mouth that was spreading, but it was a small cancer and it wasn't in my lungs or anything immense like that. It was just a small tumor! When I came back to reality, all I could think about was that God could handle this.

Though the shock of learning about my treatment was enormous, I still had perfect peace. Amid this "mother of all bombs" being dropped on my life, I continued to experience God's peace. Paul stated in Philippians 4:7, "Then you will experience God's peace, which exceeds anything we can understand. His peace will guard your hearts and minds as you live in Christ Jesus." But Paul preceded this verse with verse 6: "Don't worry about anything; instead, pray about everything. Tell God what you need, and thank him for all he has done." Now that I had done. I had prayed lots about everything I was going through. Others and I had told God about my needs, and we all thanked Him immensely for all he had done in my life and body. It was time to watch Him work.

Little did I understand at the time how greatly God had already been at work in my life through my primary care doctors, my dentist, my oral surgeons, my oncologists, my radiation oncologist, and my ENT surgeon and his great staff.

That reminds me of the old story about a man trapped in his house during a flood. To save his life, he climbed out a window onto his roof, and he prayed to God for deliverance. He was assured God would save him. A police officer came by in a boat and shouted for the man to climb down into the rescue boat. The man declined the offer. "I'm okay. God's going to save me!" The officer left. Shortly after, the fire department came along in another rescue boat and told the man to climb aboard. Once again—"I'm okay. God's going to save me!" Soon, the floodwaters grew deeper and immersed the man's home. He drowned.

He was perplexed when he came to in heaven. He told God, "Lord, I prayed and was totally convinced you'd save me!" The Lord smiled. "I tried. I sent the police and fire department to your aid, but you refused my help!"

God often uses many people to bring healing into our lives. Somedays, it goes way beyond our human understanding.

Soon after surgery, in my early days in ICU, I discovered that many of the things I thought I had had together weren't all that together. I'd thought I'd had many answers, but I discovered that my knowledge and a bunch of my pet doctrines didn't mean too much anymore. And I discovered that those doctrines weren't important anyway. I found that my healing didn't come from what I knew, believed, or confessed but from my relationship with God, my Father. He and I are one, and His ways are always higher than mine. And I soon discovered I was at peace with that.

By now, you can see that though I had not been healed by God in the way I thought I should have been healed, I was nonetheless in His perfect will and going through the healing process He had chosen for me.

> My thoughts are nothing like your thoughts, says the Lord. And my ways are far beyond anything you could imagine. For just as the heavens are higher than the earth, so my ways are higher than your ways and my thoughts higher than your thoughts. (Isaiah 55:8–9)

5

When the Miracle Doesn't Happen

Blog Post: July 13, 2016

Last fall, I was having a problem with a lower molar on the left side; it was becoming loose. My dentist told me that most likely it was dead, thus the looseness. The remedy was to pull it, which happened in late November.

Within a couple of weeks, my gums there were swelling, and I felt pressure where the tooth had been. I'd had enough teeth pulled to know what to expect, so this seemed strange. My dentist told me she'd suspected something was wrong and suggested a biopsy.

On the Wednesday before Christmas, I went to an oral surgeon for a biopsy. On January 2, the oral surgeon's office called and said I needed to get there right away. The doc told us that I had squamous cell carcinoma, a form of skin cancer that can grow in the mouth. I was referred to a local oncologist, who said that my cancer was stage 2 or most likely stage 3 and that I would need several rounds of chemo and radiation. I would also need a port surgically installed in my chest for the many IVs I would have. The process, prior to radiation, would require all my lower teeth to be extracted because no major dental work could be done for at least two years after the radiation. Having my teeth extracted before would reduce the risk of a broken jaw if they were still there and needed to be extracted from a weakened jawbone after my operation.

What I've stated above is the simple version. Amid all this, there was a lot of pain, mostly mental. I also had an ongoing battle with my insurance company, which created many delays in my treatment. However, all that time, I was expecting a miracle. As time progressed, the lower left side of my mouth was consumed by the tumor. I had severe pressure accompanied at times with uncontrolled bleeding. Once when Corrine and I were at a restaurant, my mouth suddenly began bleeding, and blood even ran out on my plate. I rushed to the men's room and began rinsing my mouth with warm water. Finally, the bleeding stopped. I left the restaurant feeling somewhat embarrassed.

I needed a miracle. Soon. Every day, I expected to feel something strange going on in my mouth ending with me spitting out the tumor. I had several people pray for that to happen, but it didn't occur.

As I write this, July 13, 2016, the seven weeks of daily radiation treatment and many rounds of chemotherapy have been completed. The tumor is probably 85 percent gone. The severe mouth sores— side effects of radiation and chemo—are about gone as well. I have a PET scan scheduled for a month from now, and we'll see where we go from there. I'm still expecting a miracle. Today very well could be the day that I spit that tumor out. Why not? Giving up is not the answer for you or me. Keep expecting your miracle, my friend, no matter what you're going through.

However, if the miracle doesn't come, please enter the place of rest that you can find only through the finished works of Christ on His cross. Remember, He said, "It is finished." He is not going to do it for you because He already has. You don't have to beg, plead, or do anything to see God do something for you.

Early on in this cancer battle, Corinne and I came to peace about seeking medical treatment and following the doctors' advice. I made it clear I didn't want to hear about how many "healing" verses I needed to confess every day. I didn't want to hear about eating certain diets, drinking certain fluids, etc. I, we, just planned on following the leading of the Holy Spirit and resting in God's love being manifested to us. The peace we both have is just out of the box. I have watched many cancer patients over the years work themselves into a frenzy trying to do everything right so they could obtain their miracle. That is works and leads only to fear, shame, and condemnation.

In the middle of this battle, Corinne and I have peace, lots of it. Of course, I want this chapter of my life to end right now. But while we wait, we have peace, boatloads of it. In all this, we have been able to obtain rest, lots of it. I continue to minister to many, and my life is getting better all the time.

But I'm not out of the woods yet. As I look back over the past several months, I see that I have changed. I'm not the same person, husband, father, or pastor I once was. I've grown in God's perfect love and acceptance, and I look forward to sharing that with many. Hey, I never want to go through this again, but it has been a good thing for me to go through. I'm seeing the lemonade God has produced from lemons. Isn't that a miracle? I believe it is.

I also believe you will obtain your miracle the moment you read this post. If it doesn't come, I'll be standing with you at your lemonade stand. Glory!

Grace and peace!

Additional Comments

In the blog post above, I mentioned that in August 2016, I was scheduled to have a PET scan to check my progress. The radiation treatments would go on for more than a month post-treatment and should have shrunk the tumor more. Though the tumor had shrunk greatly, it never totally disappeared, and just prior to the scan, the tumor began to grow. I could judge its size by the amount of pressure I felt in my mouth, which increased daily. We were stunned by how vicious and tenacious this tumor was. When people would ask me if I was in pain, I'd say, "Not really, but the pressure is very uncomfortable." I could control the discomfort with Ibuprofen, but that came with side effects.

The scan showed that the cancer had spread into the lymph nodes on the right side of my neck. The lymph nodes on the left side had already been destroyed by the radiation. My doctors were concerned, and they insisted that my insurance company approve consultation with the ear, nose, and throat department at the University of Florida, Shands Hospital. This is where the first oral surgeon, after the initial biopsy, wanted me to go in the first place! Another biopsy of the tumor was done, and within days, I was scheduled for very radical surgery, which was completed on September 15, 2016.

Corinne, I, and many others had sought God for healing, and though the miracle alluded us, we could see God's hand in the process I was about to endure. My wife and I were flooded with indescribable peace.

Family members began to fly in to be with me. The surgical waiting room was packed with my clan, which impressed the hospital staff. As Corinne and I were driving to the hospital early that morning, I was at peace. Even during surgical prep, I had no fear. This peace lasted even while I was rolling down the hall to the operating room. I even told the doctors and nurses I was at ease.

During this entire process, I was never plagued with fear, shame, or condemnation. These things wanted to attack me, but I wouldn't accept them. I knew God was working in me. I expected the miracle that never happened, but I knew my lack of the miracle was not due to my lack of faith or me being a second-class Christian. Some people suggested that my faith was lacking, but I would not receive what they were saying about me.

No two people are healed in the same way. Instead of understanding this, the church, or should I say some in the church, have transformed healing into some form of law. Remember me being afraid to take headache medication? Divine healing isn't a law or a formula or even a doctrine. Instead, it's a relationship with

God. Understanding this will form a barrier that protects us from fear, shame, and condemnation.

I learned that God wasn't healing me only of cancer; he was healing the total me. I wasn't calling Him down from heaven to set me free from sickness and disease; instead, I was acknowledging Him working in me and setting me free from my insecurities. In His prayer to the Father, Jesus said in John 17:20–21,

> I am praying not only for these disciples but also for all who ever believe in me through their message. I pray that they will all be one, just as you and I are one – as you are in me, Father, and I am in you. And may they be in us so that the world will believe you sent me.

Years ago, I discovered Christ and I were one. My bout of cancer was really His. Here's a hypothesis that may be difficult for some to grasp. For years, we have heard healing evangelists state, "Christ never was sick a day in His life, so if you fully obey Him, you won't be sick either!" I can almost see the evangelist huffing and puffing and shouting this into his microphone.

However, if Christ and I are one, it wasn't just me who had cancer, it was Christ as well. There it is. Christ went through my sickness not just *with* me but *as* me because we are one. I didn't fail God, and He didn't fail me. Instead, God, my Lover, sent His Son to go through this in me and as me. How could I lose? If you understand this, you'll never again battle fear, shame, or condemnation due to sickness.

No wonder I experienced such perfect peace that morning of surgery. It wasn't just me lying on that operating table, it was Christ as well. I was winning the battle because He was winning it in me. That gets me excited. How about you?

Once again, please read Paul's words, this time in Colossians 1:24–27.

> I am glad when I suffer for you in my body, for I am participating in the sufferings of Christ that continue for his body, the church. God has given me the responsibility of serving his church by proclaiming his entire message to you. This message was kept secret for centuries and generations past, but now it has been revealed to God's people. For God wanted them to know that the riches and glory of Christ are for you Gentiles, too. And this is the secret: Christ lives in you. This gives you assurance of sharing his glory.

I trust by now you're getting a glimpse of God's peace. In Philippians 4:6–7, we read,

> Don't worry about anything; instead, pray about everything. Tell God what you need, and thank him for all he has done. Then you will experience God's peace, which exceeds anything we can understand. His peace will guard our hearts and minds as you live in Christ Jesus.

There is no fear, shame, or condemnation in this.

6

"Larry, What's That in Your Hand?"

Blog Post: July 29, 2016

The other day, someone asked me if I was still preaching in our church. I had to tell them that since the discovery of oral cancer, I'd probably not preached more than four times in the past six months.

I am so blessed to see the people of our church share their wonderful, life-changing stories of grace while I've been unable to. I have such a wonderful church, New Covenant Grace Fellowship in Inverness, Florida. It's interesting that a preacher—me—is fighting a situation that has stopped him from talking. Of course, I'm getting a lot of the "He's going to hit us with long sermons when he gets back to preaching" wisecracks.

Here's my problem. I can't preach or teach, but the Lord keeps pouring on more intense revelations of new-covenant grace. I'm seeing so much lately that I'm asking the Lord to back off as I can't assimilate it all.

Like Moses, I sensed that the Lord asked me, "Larry, what's in your hand?" He asked that of Moses when Moses was giving his excuses to the Lord about why he couldn't be used in setting his people free from Egypt. Moses replied, "It's my rod." It was the rod that turned into a serpent when thrown to the ground and that parted the Red Sea. When God asked me that, at first, I didn't understand what He was getting at. A preacher's main tool is communication, mostly oral communication, and that's an area I currently fall short in. Speaking is painful for me, so I can't use my favorite tool. However, the Lord was showing me I could still communicate. My new rod of communication is writing. I'm being challenged to throw that rod on the ground and watch what the Lord does with it.

During this time of less oral communication, I'll be doing everything I can to share with any who are interested through written communication. The message continues to be grace and more grace. Once again, the Lord is taking my situation and turning my lemons into lemonade. Glory! I will not be silenced especially when so many are hungering for the simple truths of new-covenant grace.

Lol … That's my story, and I'm sticking to it.

Grace and peace!

Additional Comments

When I woke up after surgery in my ICU room, I was all wired up and totally disoriented. Corinne, some family members, my doctors, and some nurses were there. I tried to speak, but due to the radical surgery in my mouth and neck as well as having a trach, speaking was impossible, and that added to my confusion. I had known I would have problems talking, so before the surgery, Corinne purchased a small whiteboard and some markers for me, and I used them to communicate. I never went anywhere without my board and a marker or two.

I was bedridden in the ICU. When I was transferred to my regular room, my board came with. My only communication with Corinne, my doctors, and nurses was through that board, and Corrine even had to get more markers because I went through them quickly. Sometimes, my board would get lost in the blankets, but the nurses were very helpful in locating it. They knew it was my only form of communication, so they didn't want my board lost either.

The only nutrition I could take in was a liquid diet through a tube inserted in my stomach. At least I didn't have to order food from a menu, and at the time, eating solid food was the furthest thing from my mind. I suffered constant thirst, but I wasn't allowed to drink any water. Later, I could suck on some crushed ice. I remember writing on my board to a nurse, "I could kill for a Pepsi!" She laughed and said, "Do you want me to pour a soda down your G tube?"

I soon discovered that my whiteboard was my rod that God could use through me. It may seem like a small thing, but believe me, that whiteboard was a lifeline for me. One day, one of the nurses came into the room and said, "Your wife is so awesome the way she comes here every day to see you." I wrote, "Yes she is, and she has to drive ninety minutes each way to get here!" I wrote that our fiftieth wedding anniversary was coming up the next month. She was amazed; she said she didn't know many people who had been married that long. I wrote a few sentences about how we had almost ended in divorce years ago but that our faith in Christ had ended that. I was using my board as a ministry tool. My nurse was wiping tears from her eyes. I thought, *Lord, you're using me to lift you up and I can't even talk!*

I could write a lot more about how God used me and my board when I was hospitalized, but I want to share with you the importance of not capitulating to the dreadful things that go along with sickness and disease. Instead, pick up your rod—whatever it is—and allow the fullness of God in you to raise up His standard through you.

Those days were very difficult for me; I had to constantly fight off depression. I even had thoughts of me not being able to overcome the ordeal. I remember telling Corinne, "If I'd known how hard this would be, I'd never have agreed to the operation." A few times, very brief thoughts of suicide entered my thinking. But my ability to keep ministering to others through my board was my lifeline to reality. In the middle of that darkness, God had provided an extremely bright light for me to employ.

I still have difficulties speaking. Often, I must concentrate very carefully on how I form my words. Others say they can understand me, but I have a challenging time understanding myself. The tip of my tongue is numb, and I still deal with swelling in my mouth and neck. It sounds to me like I'm talking with marbles in my mouth. I have preached several times over the past few months, but that causes more swelling that makes speaking difficult for me for several days.

Right now, I'm in the middle of having four Sundays off in a row. The important thing, though, has been my ability to write as a tool of ministry. I use Facebook, my blog, and even this book as my rod of power.

Please don't be overcome by the darkness of your sickness and disease. Many years ago, while working full time and ministering full time, I was going through a hard place in my life. One day, I was at work on break and drinking coffee when Brother Ron walked in and yelled, "Silverman, what have you done for God today?" I was totally depressed and drowning my sorrows in my coffee; that was the last question in the world I wanted to answer, but it eventually helped me snap out of my funk. God had used a big mouth to knock me back to reality. I'm not suggesting you must work hard at doing things for God for your healing to take place; you most likely have heard enough of that legalistic nonsense. But I suggest you look within, listen to the still, small voice of God, and follow His leading. You may be surprised at what materializes despite sickness or disease.

God has not made you sick for Him to work out issues in your life. He has not placed any disease in your life so He can speak to you. It was never His will for you to be sick in the first place. These are facts, and it's imperative that you believe them. Your sickness, injury, or disease is not in the will of God period! But during it all, you can pick up the rod that God shows you and make a difference for someone even if your dark days are terminal. In the middle of your battle, you will find inner strength. Paul said in 2 Corinthians 4:17,

For our present troubles are small and won't last very long. Yet they produce for us a glory that vastly outweighs them and will last forever! So, we don't look at the troubles we can see now; rather, we fix our gaze on things that cannot be seen. For the things we see now will soon be gone, but the things we cannot see will last forever.

I eventually saw myself living in the vastness of the unseen world. I found even more peace there, and you will too!

7

Help! I Don't Have Enough Faith to Get Healed!

(Due to the nature of these blog posts, there is a lot of repetition included. I chose to allow the repetition to stand as removing it would take away from the overall effect of the blog. I trust that you understand.)

Blog Post: August 25, 2016

As I've stated before, I was told that I had cancer in my mouth the first week of January 2016. As a result, I have gone through full rounds of chemo and radiation. As of today, August 25, the tumor is still there and growing, and I have severe mouth sores as a side effect of the treatment. There is also a strong possibility that the cancer has spread to a lymph node on the other side of my neck. So here I am, a preacher who can no longer preach, at least with my mouth. I now await an appointment with a surgeon.

My wife and I felt led to and were very comfortable in seeking medical treatment for this affliction. At the same time, we believe in God for a miracle of deliverance from this cancer. I can't tell you how much prayer I have had during these days. People all over the world are praying for me. Last Sunday, a young man, the son of one of our members, was visiting our church service. As he was leaving, he gave me a huge hug and said, "Pastor Larry, I want you to know that I pray for you every day." He had tears in his eyes as he proclaimed that, and I was blown away.

I often discover through the grapevine that I'm on prayer lists all over the country. I have been anointed with oil, had people with miracle ministries pray for me, and have experienced so much laying on of hands that I've had more hair rubbed off my head. Yet thus far, the miracle I'm believing for has eluded me.

So, what have I been doing wrong? How have I failed God? Why is God angry with me? Or what lessons is He trying to teach me through all this? These are the traditional questions that old-covenant religion has taught us to ask. The fact is that none of these or any other related questions apply to me. And if you're going through a battle of health, they don't apply to you either!

I guess I've never asked God, "Lord, why me?" I've never doubted His love for me, and I've never doubted His healing virtue. Yet I'm still awaiting my miracle. So, the religious answer to my predicament must be, "I don't have enough faith to be healed." If that's my situation, my response must be that I read more "healing" scriptures, quote and confess that I am healed, command and demand that the devil takes his hands off me, and so on. All the above add up to just some more religious works. No, I haven't done any of those self-effort, legalistic tasks. Instead, even throughout my days of pain and tears and seeming faith failures, I've enjoyed the rest of God. That has been wonderful, and it's miraculous!

Here's a bold statement: God does not heal the sick based only on their faith. The TV evangelists have taught us that, but friends, it's just not the truth. Please go back with me to ancient Egypt. There, we meet two Jewish slaves, Moe and Curly. They were neighbors, and they were in Goshen when God told Moses that the last of the plagues was about to hit. This plague would be the death angel who would smite all the firstborn. God told Moses, "They are to take some of the blood and smear it on the sides and top of the door frames of the houses where they eat the animal" (Exodus 12:7). The animal was the first Passover lamb that each family was to slay and eat that night. God told His people that by doing that, they would be safe from the death angel.

Our two neighbors had gone home, prepared the meal, and applied the blood to their doors. They waited. Moe was a pillar of faith to his family. He led them in prayer and worship knowing nothing bad would happen to them. But Curly was falling apart. He was fretting, pacing back and forth, and hoping Moses had been telling the truth. Curly wasn't displaying any faith at all. What a contrast.

Of these two slaves, which one would experience greater favor with God? Whose house would the death angel pass over? The man of great faith, or the one of much lesser faith? The answer is simple—both were secure. God said, "When I see the blood, I will pass over you. This plague of death will not touch you when I strike the land of Egypt" (Exodus 12:13). This great deliverance was not dependent on Moe's or Curly's faith but on the shed blood and God's Word.

My friend, likewise, your healing, your miracle, is not dependent on what you do or don't do. It's dependent only on the blood shed for you two thousand years ago. It will come to you in the way and fashion that God decides to bring it to you because of that shed blood. All you must do is rest in the plan of God for your life.

Here's the deal—even if I'm never healed of cancer in this life, I cannot lose because I will spend eternity free of cancer and any other sickness. I'm the winner!

Kick religion out of your health situation and enter the wonderful rest of God through the finished works of Jesus Christ. You'll never be sorry.

Grace and peace!

Additional Comments

The faith issue has been kicked around the church for many years. When I was a young believer, Christian TV was in its infancy. I heard preacher after preacher stating that all we needed to fix every problem or issue in our lives was to increase our faith. One famous

TV evangelist named his ministry "Ever Increasing Faith." The message of the day, one that still lingers, was that if we had more faith, we would be healed and blessed and would prosper. These faith teachers wrote books, produced cassette tapes by the millions, and taught people that any lack in their lives resulted from their not exercising enough faith. Faith was the solution to all life's problems.

How well I remember trying to do things to increase my faith. I was told that if I prayed, fasted, read my Bible more, attended every church service, gave more money, etc., my faith would increase. But my problems remained, and I was living under fear, shame, and condemnation. I just couldn't measure up. Can you relate?

My self-effort became the answer to my problems. I started thinking I wasn't doing enough to gain God's favor that would allow Him to deliver me. Self-effort, or works, became a law for me. I constantly judged my obedience to this law by the events of my life. I thought that if I obeyed God, I would end up with His abundant blessing, and if I didn't obey Him, I would continue to live in lack. It was that simple.

Back in the day, other preachers and I would place significant importance on the simple word *if.* Many messages were preached based on Deuteronomy 28. This Old Testament chapter deals with the blessings for obedience and the curses for disobedience. We all lived in fear of that chapter. Most of us felt we must have had some secret sin in our lives, something that had caused us to live in disobedience because it seemed that everyone we knew lived under a curse from God. Our prayers were not answered. We all had lack. Many of us were sick and not healed. Many of us couldn't pay our bills though we tithed until it hurt. If we had been honest, we would have discovered that many of us were in bad marital relationships. Yes, it seemed we were cursed, so we must have been disobedient. However, we were told that if we would only improve ourselves and become more obedient, our faith would increase and our problems would cease.

Some certainly attained success in these areas; they went on to become famous TV preachers, developed huge churches, wrote books by the thousands, and produced TV shows that they needed to beg money for to keep on the air. Yet the rest of us just couldn't make it; we just couldn't increase our faith no matter how hard we tried. Because of that Old Testament chapter and its key word, *if*, we were doomed to the curse. As hard as we tried to obey, we just couldn't make it; we just didn't have enough faith.

That was because we didn't realize Deuteronomy 28 had not been written to us but to "all the people of Israel while they were in the wilderness east of the Jordan River" (Deuteronomy 1:1). I wasn't there in the wilderness along with the people of Israel in those days, were you? This old-covenant book of Law has no bearing on how God now blesses us under the new covenant. In Galatians 3:10–14, Paul stated,

> But those who depend on the law to make them right with God are under his curse, for the Scriptures say, "Cursed is everyone who does not observe and obey all the commands that are written in God's Book of the law." So it is clear that no one can be made right with God by trying to keep the law. For the Scriptures say, "It is through faith that a righteous person has life. This way of faith is very different from the way of law, which says, "It is through obeying the law that a person has life." But Christ has rescued us from the curse pronounced by the law. When he was hung on the cross, he took upon himself the curse for our wrongdoing. For it is written in the Scriptures, "Cursed is everyone who is hung on a tree." Through Christ Jesus, God has blessed the Gentiles with the same blessing he promised to Abraham, so that we who are believers might receive the promised Holy Spirit through faith.

Can you see the importance of these verses? Paul was saying that if we follow the Law of Moses or in fact any law that made us seem right with God, we were under a curse. No one can be made right with God by trying to keep a law. The life of faith is far different from a life of law.

Christ rescued us from the curse of the Law, including the curses in Deuteronomy 28. Christ on the cross took upon Himself all our wrongdoing. Through Christ, God has blessed even the Gentiles with the same blessing with which He blessed Abraham. Through Christ and our faith in Him, we receive the Holy Spirit.

This stuff is important. It's vital to us especially if we're going through any problem, including health issues. In the above verses, do you see any area where fear, shame, or condemnation can develop? I don't.

The word *faith* was used several times in these verses. Its Greek meaning is to simply believe what God says is true. In this case, Paul was saying that based on what Christ had taught him, "God has blessed us with the same blessings that He blessed Abraham with." The key words here are *has blessed*. Please note that Paul didn't suggest if we did more or obeyed more that God would bless us more. No! Paul emphatically stated that God's blessings were a done deal. All we must do to appropriate them into our lives is believe that we have them.

So, what happens if we choose not to believe we have God's blessings? The answer is simple. Remember our two Hebrew slaves from the blog post, Moe and Curly? Moe obviously believed God but Curly didn't; regardless, they were equally blessed. If I blessed every reader of my book with wire transfers of a million dollars each, all of them would become millionaires. Those who chose to believe this would check with their banks and find out they had been significantly blessed. But those who didn't believe it wouldn't bother checking with their banks and would never find out that they were indeed millionaires, and their lives wouldn't reflect their new riches.

Before you go online to check your bank balance, please

rest assured that I haven't sent you a million dollars. But I trust this illustration helps drive home my point. We've all received a million bucks—a measure of faith: "Be honest in your evaluation of yourselves, measuring yourselves by the faith God has given us" (Romans 12:3). God has given everyone faith to some degree or another. Some may think that because they're still sick, God hasn't given them enough faith to be healed. Isn't that a morbid thought? We're sick, God has given us His faith, but evidently, it's not enough faith to be healed? That doesn't describe my God. Yet we read above that through Christ, God has given us Abraham's blessings. That gift was given to us all.

My definition of the healing of cancer miracle in me was simply being able to spit out the tumor. But God's definition was for me to be far more greatly healed not just of cancer but of other issues I had in my life as well. I found rest in accepting God's definition. If I were to hold onto only my definition, I would have found my faith lacking and myself living in fear, shame, and condemnation.

As young pastors, Corinne and I planted a small church in a small Midwest town. An elderly couple eventually joined us. The wife was wheelchair bound; she had had polio at an early age, a common disease then. Her deformed feet had never grown. She would tell us of her desire to be healed by God and walk again. When she was a young woman, the famous "faith healer" of those days, Oral Roberts, was holding meetings nearby. She told her parents she wanted to go to the meetings and be healed by Brother Roberts. To demonstrate her faith, she asked her parents to allow her to purchase a new pair of shoes so that when she got up from the wheelchair, she would have shoes to wear.

As Oral Roberts prayed for her, she clutched the box of new shoes. Nothing happened. She left the meeting feeling dejected and rejected by God. What a letdown. She had done everything right, but God hadn't healed her. She told people she just hadn't had enough faith to be healed.

When she was a part of our church, she was in her early eighties.

We realized she carried a lot of hurt and bitterness that manifested itself in depression. Based on her definition of healing and apparent lack of faith, she was not healed. However, her life was plagued with far greater problems than just not being able to walk. Her potential contribution to the kingdom of God was stifled because she thought she didn't have enough faith to be healed. This sad scenario is very common in the body of Christ today. Due to their lack of faith, many live lives are driven by fear, shame, and condemnation.

God's definition of my miracle was far greater than just me spitting the tumor out. I knew that God loved me, Christ had blessed me, and nothing was based on my performance. I also knew that God had healed me two thousand years ago and that it would happen in a way only He would choose. Though fear, shame, and condemnation tried to come upon me, I could reject them. I had some close calls, but I did overcome because I knew that I had already been healed. I did receive my miracle, a special miracle designed by God just for me. I find total peace and rest in knowing this.

He has a specially designed miracle planned just for you as well. To see it, you must let go of your preconceived ideas and accept His plan for your life. Yes, you do have enough faith to be healed; He's already given it to you. Aren't you thrilled that the faith issue no longer depends on you?

8

Are You Sick? Don't Be Condemned!

[Please note: This is the last of the series of blog posts I wrote during my dark days of cancer prior to and after surgery. My desire during those days was to write far more than I did. However, due to all the complications and weakness of my body, I didn't have it in me to communicate any more than necessary. But I remained full of revelation, and my heart often broke because I just couldn't physically perform. Those days were days of rich learning. God was working in me a far greater thing than just healing me of cancer. Again, please forgive the repetition.)

Blog Post: November 1, 2016

First, allow me to say that I do believe in miracles and the healing power of God. I have witnessed too many of them over the years in those I have ministered to and myself to deny them or to say God no longer heals the sick.

However, I have witnessed a great deal of false teaching over the years that has brought those seeking miracles for their bodies into a state of fear, shame, and condemnation. Recently, someone told a member of our church that the reason people were sick in our church was because there was not enough teaching on healing. Of course, I totally reject this as the message of our church. New Covenant

Grace Fellowship in Inverness, Florida, is centered on Christ and His ministry to us in body, soul, and spirit. I believe our church is a harvest ground for miracles. Just about anything can and does happen!

However, we reject any teaching that can lead people into any form of fear, shame, or condemnation. Please remember that anytime we try to apply a law to our lives, whether it's the old- covenant Law of Moses or a law we make up ourselves that might make us think we are pleasing God more by following it, the only result can be condemnation.

Romans 8:1 is one of the most important verses in the Bible: "So now there is no condemnation for those who belong to Christ Jesus." This is how the verse applies to what I'm writing. If you're going through physical health issues and are seeking God for your healing, that's good. But if you're trying to fit some type of law or formula into this healing venture, that's alarming. Give up on that, Bunkie, as it will only lead you into condemnation.

It is possible that you may not be quoting enough healing Bible verses, or not be praying enough, or not have a totally positive confession—the list goes on. If after all this, you still are not healed, then ol' Mr. Condemnation followed by his friends, Mr. Fear and Mrs. Shame, will soon knock on your door. You'll begin hearing, "If only you were a better Christian, God would heal you." This thinking and teaching is pure trash, and you must reject it completely.

You may know of my recent bout of cancer and subsequent major surgery. That's right—I didn't receive an instant miracle. I had to go the route of medicine. However, there is not enough room to write of the miracles I received in this process. Here's one. After twelve hours of major surgery, I experienced zero pain. Also, as I recovered, I didn't suffer at all from any of those old devils—fear, shame, and condemnation. They tried to enter my life; I heard them knocking, but I didn't answer. Dealing with cancer and all its ramifications is bad enough, but to deal with fear, shame, and condemnation at the same time is much more than anyone can tolerate.

You may not be the perfect Christian. You may not be doing everything right to receive your healing, but the bottom line is that God loves you and that His love is not based on what you do or don't do. He loves you because He is Love and cannot do anything else. So, if you're sick, give up on the religious laws that some teachers would like to put you under and simply embrace the love of God. Watch and see what will happen. Condemnation kills, fear cripples, and shame is deceitful. Love, however, heals and brings life. That, my friend, is the true gospel of healing in the new covenant, and it works every time.

One last point—if you are never physically healed and you die, wow! Talk about the perfect healing. More on this subject later.

Grace and peace!

Additional Comments

As I dwell on what I wrote last November, I remember difficult and dark days. As I was going through the many battles that this ordeal brought, I had no idea just how sick I was. In those days, God's hand was on me, working in me, and providing me His perfect peace.

As I previously stated, fear, shame, and condemnation tried to attack me. However, Corinne and I strongly feel that my understanding of God's wonderful gift of new-covenant grace protected me from those attacks. I am certain that if I had still been embracing a mixed message of law and grace, most likely, I would not only have suffered fear, shame, and condemnation, but I would also have physically perished.

The miracle of having no pain was just one of the many miracles I experienced. However, pain is an important matter to discuss anytime we deal with health issues. I know how critical pain can be; I've experienced a lot of it over the years and know how distracting it can be. Even a paper cut can hurt enough to draw your attention to it, but what I'm discussing here is much greater pain.

Just within the past couple of years, I have suffered extreme gout pain. Even in the hospital, post-surgery, I had to be placed on a lower-protein liquid diet being put into my G tube to prevent gout attacks. But there was no pain from the surgery itself. Who can figure? I'd had my jaw replaced, my leg cut open so a bone could be removed, but there was no pain—none. However, if I would eat the wrong food, pain in my feet and hands could get unbearable. This situation just didn't make sense. Pain from gout but no pain from major surgery?

I was attached to a morphine pump for pain management. They would check out how much morphine I was using daily. The poor nurses were getting angry with me because they saw that my morphine levels were remaining the same. At first, they thought the equipment was malfunctioning. I recall one gal getting pretty upset at me and saying, "You just have to be using the morphine!" Later, I felt to hit the morphine button a couple of times per day just to get them off my back.

Prior to surgery, I read on the "Internet Doctors" that the pain in my leg would be extreme and could be worse than the pain in my jaw. Well, I had absolutely no pain in my jaw or leg. That, my friend, was a miracle.

The first liquid diet I was on for a few days was followed by gout pain. I texted my oldest daughter, who works in a medical library, asking her to research that liquid diet. She replied that it contained elevated levels of protein. I mentioned this to the nurses, my diet was changed, and the pain decreased. Do you see the irony? I had no pain from major surgery, but I did have ongoing gout attacks. If God can take care of the surgery pain, why not the gout? See? That's the perplexing nature of all this healing stuff.

Over the years, I have observed many people healed of one thing yet suffering from something else. I've often asked God, "What's this all about?" The answer is usually, "My ways are higher than your ways." Who can figure it? In all of this, we must just rest.

During my weeks of hospitalization, I had a lot of time to think about these things. I quickly concluded that I no longer had all the answers and that there were just some things I couldn't understand. I used to think I had this healing thing well in hand. I would stand before congregations all over the country and tell them God would heal them of every physical issue right then. Yes, I witnessed many being healed just as I stated. However, I also saw some who had been healed during the service lose that healing by the time they got to their cars in the parking lot, and others left the services not healed at all. I used to be mystified by such events. After all, Jesus told His disciples, "You shall lay hands on the sick and they shall recover" (Mark 16:18).

For years, I traveled the country proclaiming my favorite verse of scripture, "Jesus Christ is the same yesterday, today and forever" (Hebrews 13:8). I would state that if Jesus ever healed the sick before, He is healing the sick today. I totally believed that, and I still do. But as I discovered while lying in my hospital bed, there was much I just didn't understand. Again, a good example would be the gout pain I was dealing with and the total lack of pain from surgery.

I recall eating some fish for dinner on a Saturday evening a couple of years prior to this cancer battle. Within an hour, gout pain began to develop in my right elbow. By bedtime, the pain was so severe that Corinne called my doctor's answering service. I was told to immediately go to the emergency room. She, I, our daughter, and our son-in-law waited for hours for me to be treated and get some pain meds. It's possible that I had experienced the most intense pain of my life that night. For years, this terrible condition in my body had been prayed for extensively, but it had never left me. Then in the hospital, I had gout pain but no other pain. Who can figure? I still believe "Jesus Christ is the same yesterday, today and forever." I will also continue to preach that and will continue to minister healing to people whenever the need exists. I will then enter rest and leave the results to God.

I do not understand all that is involved, but I'm not ashamed to say so. Yes, I will minister to people, lay hands on them, and believe God along with them, but I know that healing is entirely up to God. It is never due to my fault or my lack of faith that some are not healed the way I think they should be, and it's not their fault either. My friend, I'm no longer ashamed to say there are some things I just don't understand. I'm not God, whose ways are much higher than mine.

Yet in all this, I encourage you to believe God for your healing miracle. Please don't give up. Instead, rest in your understanding of living fully in His arms of love.

As of today, May 3, 2017, I am completely pain free from gout issues as well. The G tube was removed about three months ago, and I've been eating normal food. I still have a problem eating some foods; I'll need my lower teeth replaced someday. Also, some food gets stuck in my mouth. Due to all the nerves in my lower jaw being removed or severed, I no longer have any feeling there. I can slobber food down my face and not be aware of it. I use a ton of napkins every time I eat. Every Sunday, several of our church gang eat lunch somewhere together. Most of them have learned to point to their mouths when they see food about to run down my face. I don't have the slightest idea that it's happening. It's rather funny now. In saying this, I am no longer on a low- protein, low-uric acid diet. I can't even remember the last time I've had a major gout attack. So, you see, even in this, healing has taken place. It certainly didn't manifest itself the way I wanted it to, but nevertheless, it's happened, and I'm thrilled!

Again, I say, "Don't give up!"

9

THE GREAT HIGH-WIRE ACT

When I was a child, the Shrine Circus would visit our town, Grand Rapids, Michigan, every year. I recall the schools used to take the afternoon off and bus the students to the civic auditorium, and we would enjoy an afternoon away from school at the circus.

I loved watching the acts, the animals, and the clowns, but my favorite was the high-wire acts. The performers would walk the whole distance and even ride bicycles across the wires. *How in the world do they do that?* I'd ask myself. Later, I realized these performers had learned to harness their ability to balance well.

I used to think about that balance thing; I wondered if I would ever be able to walk a wire. Eventually, I realized I could balance well. Maybe not good enough to walk a high wire, but I sure knew how to ride my bike. My dad taught me that. He said, "Once you learn how to ride a bike, you will never forget how to do it." Though I haven't ridden a bike in many years, I'm certain I could manage to ride it down our road and eventually, with a little practice, do so respectably. Once you learn balance, you never forget it. The circus performers had the balance thing under control.

For years, I have thought that one of the key lacking ingredients within the Church of today is balance. I first placed my trust in Christ in 1973. Since then, I have observed many pet movements come and go; if you have been in the Church a while, you've seen your share as well. It appears that some new thing is taught and everyone claims it as the new answer to God's blessings on their lives. People seem so desperate these days; they firmly hold onto every new thing that might offer them relief from their dilemmas. Before long, an out-of-balance state occurs with a new law that if followed brings God's blessings. Remember what we've stated—following a law always leads to fear, shame, and condemnation.

I feel that divine healing teachings in the church have gotten out of balance. I base that on many years of experience in the healing ministry and having observed the lives of many in the body of Christ. It seems that many have turned healing into a law that causes people to fall off the high wire right into fear, shame, and condemnation.

Here are some words of Jesus that a few faith preachers don't want you to read: "Here on earth you will have many trials and sorrows. But take heart, because I have overcome the world" (John 16:33). During my recovery time from surgery, I had to deal with "many trials and sorrows." I ended up with several complications that manifested themselves because of all the treatment.

My neck was severely cut just under my chin so all my lymph nodes there could be removed. Some of the nodes were cancerous, and the remaining ones came out as a precaution. That resulted in a great deal of swelling in my neck. I still have some disfigurement and swelling below my chin.

Shortly after arriving home from my long hospital and rehab stay, a fistula opened in my neck. I was amazed about how much infection came out of that thing. Later, I had two more form. After the first one opened, I had to be readmitted into the hospital for four days. After my extended stay, the last place in the world I wanted to be was back in the hospital.

Soon, Corinne was taught how to pack the fistulas by pushing a long length of treated ribbon a quarter inch wide into the hole twice daily. In the initial stages, she would put about three or four feet of ribbon into the hole. Thankfully, I had no feeling under my neck, so there was no pain involved, just a strange sensation. After about three weeks, the holes would close and the packing would end.

Another side effect of the surgery was severe sleep apnea. Due to being overweight, I had had some sleep apnea issues prior to surgery. Corinne would tell me that some nights when I would stop breathing, she would give me a shove to get me to breathe again. But post-surgery, this became a very significant issue. It was not caused by my weight; by that time, I had lost many pounds. However, anytime I fell asleep, even sitting in a chair and during any time of the day or night, I would stop breathing and would awake startled and gasping for air. This developed during the last days of my hospital stay and increased after I arrived home. I was dealing with a fistula and not breathing during sleep as well. At one point, I couldn't sleep at all for about three days.

The most demanding thing I had to deal with was the tracheotomy. I needed a tube inserted into my lower neck so I could breathe during and immediately after surgery. It was a constant irritant especially as I was healing speedily. I can remember the choking sensation that it constantly caused. Soon after I moved to my regular room from ICU, Dr. Boyce told me that when I could breathe for twenty-four hours with the trach capped, he would remove it. What a frustrating struggle that process was. I had to place a plastic cap over the opening of the trach and breathe normally through my mouth and nose. At first, I could keep it capped for only an hour or so. That was very discouraging; I wanted that thing out.

One time, I went for about eleven hours with the cap on, but then I just stopped breathing, so I had to quickly pull the cap off. Because of the trach, I had to be transported from the main hospital to the Shands Rehab Hospital by ambulance. Corinne was not allowed to take me by car because I needed medical staff with me in case I stopped breathing.

Once I was in rehab, the doctor there told me that once I could keep the cap on for forty-eight hours, he would remove the trach.

"Wait! Dr. Boyce told me I needed only twenty-four hours!" I had to fight a little on that deal. Finally, rehab called Dr. Boyce, and they agreed to twenty-four hours. I did it, and that silly thing was removed. What a great victory that event was!

I share these three difficulties with you to relate how my life fit what Jesus meant when He said, "Here on earth you will have many trials and sorrows." The King James Version calls these trials and sorrows *tribulation*. Yet thankfully, the balance to these words is, "But take heart, because I have overcome the world." We must face the fact that dreadful things happen to good people. But it is also factual that Jesus Christ has overcome the world. The Overcomer lives in us, so we too overcome the world. I overcame the above complications and several more because I am an overcomer. Christ abides in me, and He lives in you too.

This is how I now see the healing thing—God is my healer. Christ lives in me. He shed His blood for me. I received healing two thousand years ago. Christ in me conquered sickness and disease. God still performs miracles. I am ready to receive miracles of healing. I expect to be healed, but I may not be. If I am not healed and go through trials and sorrow, Christ still lives in me. Because Christ lives in me, I will overcome any trials or sorrows I may face. I am an overcomer! There's a lot of balance in those statements. By following this mind-set, I am free from any law leading to fear, shame, or condemnation.

In life, we often find ourselves walking a high wire. But when we do, we must remember that Christ has overcome our world. No matter what comes our way, we can overcome. We don't do this alone under our own power; if we try that, we'll fail. Instead, we overcome by the power of God in us and knowing He loves us. No matter what complications we face, our Healer remains in us. If we see healing manifested in our situation, we can praise God. If we don't see healing manifested, even if we face death itself, we can still praise God. He is in charge, and knowing, living, and experiencing that brings great peace even amid life's worst storms.

We never need to fear falling off the high wire because Christ is our balance. Once we learn that, we'll never forget it.

10

Positive Confession—Yes or No?

As I write this book, I'm overwhelmed by the numbers of friends I have who need a healing touch from God. It seems that so many are going through difficult battles these days. Maybe I'm more aware of cancer now, but it seems to me that cancer is running wild.

Since my personal contact with cancer, I've had the opportunity to think about my childhood. I can't remember too many people having cancer then. I remember my aunt passing away from cancer, but that's about it. Even in our family circle of friends, we hardly ever heard of people dying because of cancer. Wow! How things have changed. It seems that lately, everyone I know is being affected by cancer in one way or the other. Something has certainly changed.

When I was living my dark days of active cancer, many friends would encourage me to write a book about my journey. I agreed because I felt God had put another book in my heart, but I just didn't have the physical energy to do it. So, I managed to postpone writing a book until better days arrived. I'm sure that the timing wasn't right then; I was enmeshed in the healing process of my entire person—spirit, soul, and body. However, now I'm feeling compelled to get this book written, published, and released because I sense strongly that many people need to read what I am writing.

Most likely, you picked up this book because you needed it

yourself or you knew a friend or relative who was struggling with sickness and disease. Maybe you will feel led to pass this book on to someone who needs it more that you do. My hope and prayer is that you or whoever reads this book will be encouraged by my journey into divine health. Certainly, this story is mine. However, my desire is that somehow through these words, you too will find total healing and peace. My longing is for your story to end as well as mine has.

The questions always seem to arise, "How important is my positive confession? Is a positive confession, the words we speak out of our mouths, vitally essential for God to heal us?" My response deals with definitions. I don't believe a positive confession is necessary or vital for God to heal anyone. I realize this is not what "faith healers" would teach.

Several years ago, Corinne and I lived and traveled full time on the road ministering in churches all over America. Our only home was a thirty-seven-foot motor home named Pilgrim 1. We experienced a lot during those days. Maybe one day I'll write a book about those times of travel and ministry.

We noticed that people who held to the teaching of certain faith preachers were the hardest to minister to and the last to ever be healed. I'm sure you too find this fact interesting. Often, we would preach or teach in a meeting and then call the people up for personal ministry. Many times, they would stand in a line; Corinne and I would lay hands on them, pray for their needs, and speak positive words into their lives. We often noted that some people seemed to receive this ministry simply but others seemed to be resistant and closed off to what we felt God wanted to do in their lives.

Those who adhered to what we called hyper faith were the most difficult to minister to. We would often ask them, "What would you like God to do for you?" Most likely, their response would be something like, "I don't want to tell you what I need because I don't want to confess something negative." Sometimes, they would expect us to know exactly what they needed. Occasionally, we did know what certain people needed prior to ministering to them, but most of the time, we didn't.

It seemed to us that these people possessed a haughtiness, something that defied what we were trying to accomplish for them. One night in a hotel meeting in Pennsylvania, the wife of a tall, young man helped him into the meeting room and found a seat for him. I could see he was in great pain. We had a worship team leading the meeting, and when they were done, I received the microphone. I was about to begin my message when I was strongly drawn to the young man who was obviously hurting. I believed the Holy Spirit was directing me to pray for this guy right away, even before I brought my message. I walked to him and asked if I could pray for him. As I began ministering to him, I could see pain immediately leaving his body. I didn't pray a long, drawn-out prayer but a rather short one, but by the time I was done, all the pain had left. As I often did in situations like this, I asked him to try to do what he couldn't do before ministry. He began jumping and rapidly bending over to touch his toes. All pain had left him. He had received a miracle healing! I was excited, and so was everyone else there. Everyone's faith was running strong.

Right next to this guy was an elderly woman to whom I was drawn. I noticed that her fingers were badly twisted. I realized she was suffering from severe rheumatoid arthritis. Nevertheless, I asked her what the Lord could do for her that night. Her smug answer was, "Oh, nothing. I was healed two thousand years ago, and I'm only confessing that!" I perceived arrogance in her words. I asked about the arthritis in her hands, and she said she didn't have arthritis any more though it was obvious she did. I asked if I could pray for her anyway, and she agreed. However, I sensed that if I prayed for the wall of the building next to her, I'd experience more acceptance. She went home with the arthritis still showing in her hands.

Her positive confession had become a form of a law. Her rigid concept of faith most likely had blocked her from God healing her that night. Of course, I can't know that for certain, but I felt God had pointed her out to me so she could receive a miracle.

Keeping the balance discussion from the previous chapter in mind, I say there is a place for keeping our confession, the words that come out of our mouths, positive. In the book of James, the author drew a lot of attention to our tongues. James 3:5–6 states, "In the same way, the tongue is a small thing that makes grand speeches. But a tiny spark can set a great forest on fire. And the tongue is a flame of fire. It is a whole world of wickedness, corrupting your entire body." In its proper context, this verse is speaking to people who use their words to hurt one another. However, it's also depicting just how strong the tongue can be. I stated before that I would often speak to my body things like, "My body can't ever be afflicted by cancer" or "If cancer is in my body, I command that it die and harmlessly pass from me!"

During my radiation treatments, I would lie on the table with the machine scanning the left side of my lower jaw and neck. During the treatment, I'd say, "I command cancer to die in my body and harmlessly leave me in the name of Jesus!" I would often speak these same words during my shower. Did these words work for me? I don't know, and I never will know. It may seem that my words fell off the radiation table or went down the shower drain, but who knows? It's possible that these positive words had a positive effect on the cancer that tried to eliminate me. Those positive confessions certainly never caused me any harm. However, I never made such positive words a law in my life. If I had, I would have most likely thought, *I didn't remember to speak to cancer in my body today. I must do it right now or I may really get afflicted with a dreadful case of cancer!*

Even after my cancer diagnosis, I often commanded it to die in my body. I put my finger in my mouth on top of the tumor and cursed it, commanding it to die. Did it die? No. At least not in the way I thought it should. But it did eventually die, and it's no longer in my body. So, did telling the cancer to die do any good? I believe it did. But I never came under the law of speaking to the cancer. God is my Healer, not my words. Yet the words I speak are very important to my total well-being.

My Grandpa Silverman would take me out fishing when I was young. Oh how I loved that man. I think the main reason he would take me fishing so often was that I was the only one who would go with him. My dad would never go with Gramps because he would get in a boat, throw out the anchor, and fish in one place all day even if the fish weren't biting. We would sit there holding onto old-fashioned cane poles watching our bobbers for hours on end. I loved it. I guess what I really loved was being with him.

However, one thing I didn't like about him was his confession about himself. Whenever anyone asked him "Sam, how are you doing today?" his reply was, "Pretty good for an old man." He always called himself an old man. I didn't like that because I never considered him an old man at all.

In a couple of weeks, I will become seventy. I never call myself an old man. I never will even if I live into my nineties. Despite the cancer battle that has taken a toll on my body, I don't consider myself an old man.

When I turned sixty, Laura, my daughter-in-law who works with elderly people, said, "Sixty is the new forty." I think seventy is the new fifty; that's how I feel. My battle with cancer has left me with more limitations. I find it more difficult to walk as a result all the chemotherapy along with neuropathic side effects in my hands and right foot. I may need more help getting my bass boat out and covered up again at the dock, but I do go fishing and have no plans to stop. I've slowed down, but I don't consider myself or call myself an old man.

When my dad was my age, he was constantly in pain due to arthritis in his hips; he had one replaced twice. He always told me, "Larry, it's rough getting old!" and "Whatever you do, don't get old!" I know that he spoke those words from the standpoint of great pain and suffering, but I wish he'd never called himself old. Negative words do have a negative effect.

Soon, my beautiful mother will be ninety-three. She lives by herself and still gets out some especially with the help of my wonderful sister and brother-in-law. She hurts a lot. She used to talk about her aches and pains, but lately, she seems so positive. I like that, and I expect her to be around for a long time yet. My health battle was very hard on her especially since I live in Florida and she lives in Michigan. But she overcame her fears for me just as I did. I could often feel her heartfelt prayers.

So, my friend, go ahead and make positive confessions. Declare your healing. Declare your health. If you sense that the Lord would have you march around your house three times per day declaring an end to the sickness or disease afflicting you, by all means do it. But please don't do it just because someone told you to. Speak positive confessions over your circumstances and situations; you have nothing to lose by doing so; just don't make a law of it. If you do, you're making a way for fear, shame, and condemnation to arrive.

Listen to the words of Jesus in Mark 11:22–24.

> Have faith in God. I tell you the truth, you can say to this mountain, "May you be lifted up and thrown into the sea," and it will happen. But you must really believe it will happen and have no doubt in your heart. I tell you, you can pray for anything, and if you believe that you've received it, it will be yours.

Please don't be condemned by these words. If you have been ill and are expecting a miracle, don't think your lack of faith is causing God to not heal you. First, Jesus isn't speaking about literal mountains here. Second, the emphasis here is on "Have faith in God." Trust God; He knows what He is doing and has your life under His control no matter what it looks like.

In all circumstances, we should speak to our mountains. Our words have authority. If our thoughts about God are healthy, if our thoughts about ourselves are healthy, we will speak healthy words; they will reflect what is in our hearts. However, never lose sight of the fact that God is your Healer, not your words. Also, it isn't entirely the words that you speak that make you sick either.

Avoid law at all cost. Rest in God's abundant love for you. You are in His hands. If you are healed by a God-given miracle, I say, "Glory!" On the other hand, if the miracle alludes you and you ultimately pass away, I still say, "Glory!" You can't lose. You really can't.

I spent a lot of time speaking to my mountain. Somedays, I couldn't do it, especially when I was going through challenging times. But during those times, I sensed others were carrying me, were speaking forth words of faith for me. It's important to keep positive people in your camp. I think that by now, you can understand that. I still have a challenging time when I speak. People say they can understand me, but I must work hard at forming my words. Sometimes, the proper word just isn't formed right when I say it. I sound the worst to myself; to me, I sound like I have several marbles in my mouth when I talk. When I laugh and preach, I tend to spit on people. A great deal of saliva forms when I talk a lot. That is a miracle, as several saliva glands were killed during radiation and others were removed during surgery, yet the spit sure flows when I'm preaching. I call it my miracle spit! We all have a good laugh over that during my messages. So, I find speaking to my mountain interesting as my ability to speak has been restored, not like I want and not like it will be one day, but I can speak.

You are in God's hands too. You have something positive to say about your situation in life, so go ahead and speak it! You just may be surprised by what comes out of your mouth.

11

Why Did I Get Sick?

The big question remains—Why did I get sick? The larger answer is, I don't know. How is that for dodging the issue?

Soon after surgery, having much time on my hands to think, I came upon the great discovery that many of the answers to the great theological questions of life, questions I thought I had the answers to, no longer held water. I also discovered that I had great inner peace by admitting to myself and others that I no longer had all the answers. I found it very comforting to be able to tell people, "I don't know why I got sick!"

As soon as I was diagnosed with cancer, Corinne and I felt led to go public with the condition and be honest with people. Years ago, while under the law of healing—man-made rules and regulations about health and well-being—I would have hidden the fact that my body was plagued by cancer. After all, I was God's man of power for the hour! To admit to sickness and disease was to admit to lacking faith. That meant my weakness was exposed to those I was ministering to. I was supposed to be a pillar of faith to those weaker than me.

I find that many preachers are dishonest with those they minister to by not exposing their own weaknesses; that's disturbing. Years ago, I decided that the best and most effective way of ministry is to be transparent with those I minister to. I was no better than they were, and hiding the problems in my life wasn't being fair to them. If I expose a weakness in my life, it affords me a greater opportunity to minister to the weakness in others' lives. God has given me great freedom in this area, so I felt free to say I don't know why cancer came knocking on my door.

Yes, there can be problems with transparency. When one is transparent with others, especially someone like me who has many people observing my every move worldwide, I run the risk of opening myself to all types of opinions, ideas, criticisms, and doctrines that others want to share with me so I might be healed. Therefore, from the onset, I told people that we had a course of action we felt was the right one for us to follow and that I wasn't interested in anyone's great ideas.

As a pastor and minister for many years, I have witnessed dozens, maybe hundreds of people suffer the ravages of cancer. I can't begin to count the many who had refused professional medical treatment because they read somewhere that doctors and pharmaceutical companies were becoming very wealthy due to their promotion of cancer treatments. Some believed that if they ate the proper diet, especially cancer-fighting foods, their healing would come. Others believed that smelling the right oils would cure cancer. Some even suggested that cancer could be cured by taking certain natural herbs. Others might suggest doing all the above and quoting the right Bible "healing verses" to be healed.

I cannot recall one person who was healed by doing these things and refusing medical attention. They're all dead! I also find such practices non-scriptural. Have you ever read in the four Gospels Jesus saying to someone who approached Him seeking healing, "Just eat the right foods, take the prescribed herbs, smell the proper oils, quote Bible verses, and you will be healed"? No! Jesus supernaturally healed them just as they were. Therefore, I find today's model of Jesus plus us doing something is not in the Bible.

I did try to eat better; that just made sense. Thanks to a special friend, I roll frankincense oil on my chin several times daily; it's supposed to help fight cancer. I don't know if that's true, but I like the smell. I think using common sense in these areas is important.

I told people who often were caring and had my best interests at heart, "Thank you for your idea, but I know the road to travel." Sometimes, that wasn't received well. Some became offended and felt I was rejecting them personally, not just their ideas for my healing. However, most of my family and friends respected my wishes and allowed me to go forward on my chosen road.

A man I knew recently passed away from cancer. A faith preacher said he would not survive cancer because he had chosen to believe the doctor's report instead of the Word of God. Can't you see the healing laws being set up in this scenario? Thankfully, the man with cancer was beginning to understand the wonderful message of God's grace; he didn't accept the preacher's words and avoided succumbing to fear, shame, and condemnation. He died in total peace.

However, many find themselves in such situations swallowing that preacher's condemnation hook, line, and sinker. I too have found some—very few but some—who think the same of me. "If Larry didn't believe the doctor's report and instead believed God's Word about healing, he would have been healed of cancer." Such thinking is nonsensical.

In 2 Timothy 4:3, Paul told Timothy,

> For a time is coming when people will no longer listen to sound and wholesome teaching. They will follow their own desires and will look for teachers who will tell them whatever their itching ears want to hear. They will reject the truth and chase after myths.

So many teachings today are myths; they aren't based on sound teaching. As I have stated before, I have seen too many miracle healings take place to ever doubt God still heals the sick. However, I have also seen very many children of God who have fallen prey to fear, shame, and condemnation because someone told them they were sick because they chose to believe what the doctors told them and not what the Bible said. I trust that this book is bringing some balance and reality back into the thinking of those who read it.

Did the devil make me sick? No. The devil didn't make me sick, and the devil hasn't made you sick either. I know that we look for reasons for sickness and disease; we don't want to take any blame for it ourselves. But God didn't make me sick, and neither did the devil. Then who did? Could it be that life itself made me sick? I've used a cell phone for many years and have done so extensively. Corinne and I don't have a landline. Ever since I first used a cell phone, I've held it up to my left ear especially while driving. Over the years, I've used my drive time as my talk time. I drove the car or our motor home that we drove all over the country with my right hand and held the cell phone up to my left ear with my left hand. Guess what part of my face the phone covers when I'm talking? You got it—right over the area where the tumor developed. Did I get cancer because of years of cell phone use? Maybe. I guess I'll never know, but the possibility exists. Did the devil make me hold the cell phone up to my left ear? Do I even have to answer that question?

My friend, we live in a fallen world. Our parents and grandparents were never exposed to many things that are normal for us. Look at all the processed food we eat. Just an hour ago, Corinne and I arrived home from grocery shopping, and just about every food item we purchased came in a box, can, or plastic bag. Back in the day, when I was a kid working on a neighbor's dairy farm, every summer, the corn crop was cultivated several times during the growing season to eradicate the weeds. Today's farmer wouldn't think about wasting all the fuel necessary in cultivating cornfields; instead, he just sprays an herbicide on the emerging weeds. Does cancer come from this practice? Who knows? Maybe the devil inspires the farmers of today to use herbicides instead of cultivating for weed control. I don't mean to be flippant here, but I just can't resist it.

Sickness and disease can come from many sources we aren't aware of, but to blame it all on the devil is insanity. That's because the devil is totally defeated. The only power the devil has is the power we give him or allow him to have. Here are a few verses of scripture that depict our defeated foe.

- Romans 16:20a: "The God of peace will soon crush Satan under your feet."
- Colossians 1:13: "For he has rescued us from the kingdom of darkness and transferred us into the Kingdom of his dear son."
- Colossians 2:15: "In this way, he disarmed the spiritual rulers and authorities. He shamed them publicly by his victory over them on the cross."
- Hebrews 2:14–15: "Because God's children are human beings—the Son also became flesh and blood. For only as a human being could he die, and only by dying could he break the power of the devil, who had the power of death. Only in this way could he set free all who have lived their lives as slaves to the fear of dying."

The above verses, granted taken out of context, do support the thought that the devil is a defeated foe. My purpose in this book is not to debate the power of the devil. I understand that some will disagree with my thinking that the devil didn't have the power to give me cancer. However, my point is that as for me and only me, I did not get cancer because the devil gave it to me. I have total peace in thinking that way.

I believe I live under the finished works of the cross. The last words of Jesus in John 19:30 were, "It is finished!" By His death on the cross, Jesus ended all bondages that were ever placed on human beings. There, His death ended sin, sickness, disease, and all forms of fear, shame, and condemnation. In His eyes, the cancer that ravaged my body was defeated. That is why I could win the battle over it. Yes, I was expecting the miracle of spitting the tumor out, but my miracle didn't come that way. Nonetheless, it did come! I was healed of cancer. I was delivered from horrible sickness, and as the result of it happening the way it did, I became a better person. I believe what happened to me was far more beneficial to me than just spitting the tumor out.

So why did I get sick? I just don't know. But I do know I didn't get sick because of anything I knowingly did. I didn't get sick because of anything God did. I didn't get sick because of anything the devil did. I guess it doesn't matter to me why I got sick. The question "Why did this happen to me?" just doesn't matter to me anymore. The fact is that I did get sick but am not sick any longer. God healed me, and that's all that matters to me!

12

My Guardian Angels

My post-surgery days were probably the most difficult days of my life. A few weeks prior to the operation, my surgeon, Dr. Boyce, told Corinne and me what we could expect from the operation. We were shocked. Later, I explored my upcoming operation on the Internet and was even more shocked. However, nothing really prepared me for all I experienced.

The first thing I remember after coming out of the twelve-hour procedure was seeing doctors and nurses surrounding me along with my wonderful bride, Corinne. I was very confused. I guess there were other family members in the room, but I don't remember. I couldn't speak. I remember attempting to talk, but nothing would come out of my mouth. I had my whiteboard, but I didn't think I could figure out how to use it very well.

I was breathing through a trach. I had all varieties of wires and tubes attached. I had a huge, black boot on my right foot and leg. The machines were all making noise. Three surgeons had had to work on me to get a bone out of my leg and into my jaw and do the same with a large section of my flesh to form a flap in my mouth. They had to monitor that closely to make sure blood was flowing through it. So, I was hooked up to a Doppler monitoring device; if it made noise, that meant the blood was flowing through my flap properly. If the noise stopped, I was in trouble. All of this made me feel like a man from outer space.

During my better than two weeks' stay in the hospital and in rehab, I battled some depression most likely due to the physical trauma of the procedure as well as from the medications I was on. Here again, God kept me. The depression would come and go, but it seemed to improve daily.

Depression often accompanies sickness and disease. Often, people dealing with it suffer from bad feelings about God. Again, I say depression has nothing to do with God's love for you or His acceptance of you.

From September 15th to the 23rd, I had the operation, spent five days in ICU, and was placed in a regular hospital room in Florida's Shands Hospital. Originally, we were told that my regular hospital stay would be three weeks followed by a week of rehab. However, God had a better plan. He was restoring me so quickly that the normal hospital stay was only eight days. The doctors and nurses were excited about my very rapid recovery and restoration.

On September 24, I rode in an ambulance to the University of Florida's Shands Rehab Hospital; I was there for five days. All this time, I was surrounded by praying people. I made many new friends at both locations, people I'll never forget. These staff members helped form my band of guardian angels.

My homecoming was glorious. But within a couple of days, due to severe swelling in my neck, sleep apnea began to rage. For several days, I was not able to get any sleep. Within seconds after I'd fall asleep, I would stop breathing and gasp for air. It didn't make any difference with my sleeping position either. Even riding in the car, if my head would nod and I would fall asleep, I would immediately stop breathing.

After a few days of that, I had to go back to the emergency room to be examined. A scope went up my nose and down my throat to my voice box. That was not a fun experience, but it's one I have, even to this day, to go through with follow-up exams. The lack of sleep enhanced my feelings of discouragement, which were tough feelings to fight. I told Corinne that if I had known how difficult recovery would be, I wouldn't have gone through with the surgery. Looking back, though, I'm very grateful I did go through with it.

Several days later, the swelling in my neck greatly increased. I developed choking sensations and the dry heaves. One morning, the swelling was extremely bad. I had to get up from bed. I was watching TV in our family room and suddenly had a case of the dry heaves. I looked down and discovered that my shirt was covered with a very nasty-smelling fluid. I looked again and saw the fluid was pouring from my neck. I got into the bathroom as soon as possible and grabbed a hand towel to stop the drainage. I woke Corinne so she could find me another towel as the first one was soaked.

As soon as the Doctor Boyce's office was open, she called, and we headed back to Shand's ER. I learned I had the first of what eventually would be three fistulas—holes in my neck filled with drainage. Thankfully, only the first one was infected. But I was admitted to the hospital for three more days. That was so discouraging. Going back in for another hospital stay was not my idea of fun, though I had no choice.

The fistulas had most likely been caused by the previous radiation treatments weakening the tissue of my neck, thus allowing the holes to form. To treat the fistulas, ribbon soaked in a chlorine bleach solution was pushed and packed into the opening. At first, it took nearly four feet of ribbon to fill the opening, and that had to be done twice daily. Slowly, the openings closed from the inside out and were eventually sealed. As they were healing, the amount of ribbon it took to pack the hole became less. When it got down to an inch or so, we could stop the packing.

Thankfully, due to the surgery, I had no feeling in my neck, so I didn't experience any pain even with all that packing. I underwent several weeks of daily hyperbaric oxygen treatments at our local hospital's wound center. I entered a special chamber and breathed oxygen at an elevated pressure for ninety minutes at a time. These treatments eventually strengthened the tissue in my neck by increasing blood flow to the affected area and eventually ended the fistula problem.

After another three days, I got out of the hospital. A home health care nurse came three days per week to check on the fistula and my general progress. Corinne became my chief nurse. She learned how to treat and bandage my right leg.

A couple of weeks after the first fistula was closed, another opened. That time, there was no infection, so I wasn't hospitalized. However, I did have to visit Dr. Boyce, my ENT surgeon. That was when he told Corinne that she would have to learn how to pack the fistula. She reluctantly took a lesson from him.

Later, when the third fistula opened, we didn't bother to call the doctor because she knew what to do. During a subsequent checkup, we told him about the third fistula; Corinne said she hadn't called him since she'd known how to handle it. Dr. Boyce's reply was, "When did you graduate from nursing school?" We all had a good laugh!

I wanted to share all the above with you so you'll have a better understanding of my journey. During this time, I was surrounded by those I call my guardian angels, my wonderful caregivers including my primary care medical staff, my oncologist's staff, my radiation oncologist's staff, all the doctors and nurses at UF, and the staff at Citrus Memorial Hospital's Wound Care/Hyperbaric Oxygen treatment center.

My primary angel was the most awesome, wonderful wife any man could ever have. Corinne never missed a day visiting me in the hospital. She's not a fan of freeway driving, but she never hesitated to make the hour-plus drive on I-75 between our home and Gainesville. Every night while I was in the hospital and in rehab, prior to bed time, she would call me and pray for me. Though I couldn't talk very well, her conversations and prayers for me were the high point of the day.

One night around 9:00 while I was in rehab, my room phone

rang. A nurse happened to be in my room, so she answered it. She handed me the phone and said I needed to hear what the person on the phone was saying. A nurse in Dr. Boyce's office said the pathology reports had arrived and she couldn't wait until morning to tell me that the tests indicated all the cancer had been eliminated. I began to weep at the news, and the nurse there did as well. The angels were sure ministering to me that night!

After I arrived home from the second hospital stay, due to fistula number one, another angel blessed me. We decided to call a friend of ours, a retired RN, to see if he would look in on me from time to time just to check on my progress. He immediately came over; he lived just a short distance from our house. He checked the fistula and gave Corinne some tips on packing it. He also checked the leg wound and helped her dress it. Ritchie came over twice daily thereafter. Every morning, he would show up at 9:00, and every evening, he came at 8:00. One morning, he grabbed my hand while I was still in my bed and said with tears in his eyes, "Larry, I pray for you every day." What an angel that guy is!

Years ago, during what I would call my "religious" days, I was taught that the medical profession was pretty much to be avoided by any Christian who was truly serving God and walking by faith. The condemnation I felt for having to buy pain medication for that headache I mentioned earlier persisted over the years and even dramatically increased. I'd say, "Doctors only practice medicine!" and then talk about my true Healer, Dr. Jesus. It seemed that back in those days, we were taught that doctors were the enemies of Christians living by faith. I fully believe that Dr. Jesus is my Healer in Chief. However, He is surround by a huge, great, awesome staff of other healers, the medical professionals and caregivers, my guardian angels.

Some people think going to a doctor shows a lack of faith. They think that if they choose medical treatment, they void their faith and God can't heal them. What a fallacy! I do know that some thought less of me because I sought treatment from doctors. As we entered this cancer battle, Corinne and I felt we were headed in the proper direction by seeking God's healing while being treated by doctors. We are still convinced we did the proper thing.

A man God used to write the book of Luke and the book of Acts was a medical doctor. In 1 Timothy 5:23, Paul told Timothy, "Don't drink only water. You ought to drink a little wine for the sake of your stomach because you are sick so often." Paul didn't say, "Now pray and believe God for your healing, Timothy." He was to take wine, a type of medicine of the day, for his stomach issues. I sure don't want to try to create theological doctrine from the above sketchy Bible examples, but God does work through doctors, hospitals, and medicine. Whoever designed the surgery performed on me had to have been divinely inspired by God to do so. Only God could put it in the heart and mind of a person how to correct mouth and jaw cancer by replacing the jawbone with the small bone of the leg. God had to have inspired this procedure.

Please don't think that you're a failure in God's eyes if you seek medical treatment for any sickness or disease. Please don't be afraid of medical treatment either. God uses the medical profession in His treatment of humanity. Good doctors will always acknowledge God in their treatment. I for one am very thankful for the medical treatment I received. It wasn't too many years ago that my condition would have ended my life. Certainly, God could have healed me with a miracle, but he chose another way, and I'm grateful.

Don't forget what we discussed earlier about making a law and trying to follow it. Only fear, shame, and condemnation can follow because these types of laws cannot be fully obeyed. Therefore, please resist the temptation to become legalistic about your health needs. Have an open mind about whatever types of treatment seem to avail themselves to you. God is working on your behalf; allow Him to move in your life in any way He desires. I tell people to pray for healing and expect the miraculous to occur, but at the same time, seek help. God will not reject your faith if you visit a doctor.

My friend, God is madly in love with us. He knew us from the beginning of time and has our future planned. Sometimes, our lives are plagued with setbacks and obstacles that can include sickness and disease. Yet amid these roadblocks, God is working on our behalf.

Yes, the healing you have expected from Him may not have arrived yet. It many never arrive in the manner you think it should, but it will eventually arrive in one form or another, and it will show up at the proper time. You are not a second-class Christian. You have the right amount of faith. You are not being punished or judged. Instead, you are a special person loved by Him without measure. No matter what you are going through, God loves you.

You too will be surrounded by guardian angels. God will send them to you at just the right time. Who knows? You might even encounter a real angel or two as well.

One passage in scripture has always intrigued me—2 Corinthians 4:17–18.

> For our present troubles are small and won't last very long. Yet they produce for us a glory that vastly outweighs them and will last forever. So, we don't look at the troubles we can see now: rather, we fix our gaze on things that cannot be seen. For the things we see now will soon be gone, but the things we cannot see will last forever.

My guardian angels helped me see things from an eternal point of view that I could never have seen with my natural eyes. To all my angels, I say, "Thank you. You're the greatest. May God bless you all!"

13

Everyone Ignores These Bible Verses

For me, Hebrews 11 is one of the most exciting chapters of the Bible. Though no one knows who the true author was, it is very Pauline to my way of thinking. If Paul wasn't the author, I'm certain someone very familiar with him and his teachings was.

The book seems to have been written to Jewish believers, most likely those living in Jerusalem just prior to its conquest by Titus in AD 70. I find all this information very interesting and exciting, but all the background of this epistle is diminished by the vital importance of its message. I consider Hebrews and Romans masterpieces of vital, new-covenant theology.

When I ponder this book, I'm tempted to go off the subject, but I must draw your attention to the famous chapter 11. Probably more Christian sermons have been preached based on this chapter than on any other chapter in the Bible. This chapter has been called the Roll Call of Faith. In this chapter, Paul (Oops! I mean the author) wrote about the faith of Abel, Enoch, Noah, Abraham, Sarah, Isaac, Jacob, Joseph, Moses, the people of Israel, Rahab, Gideon, Barak, Samson, Jephthah, David, Samuel, and all the prophets. God gave promises to these Old Testament men and women, heroes of faith. Some saw God partially fulfill His promise during their lifetimes, but most didn't. It is said of them,

> All these people died still believing what God had promised them. They did not receive what was promised, but they saw it all from a distance and welcomed it. They agreed that they were foreigners and nomads here on earth. Obviously, people who say such things are looking forward to a country they can call their own. They were looking for a better place, a heavenly homeland. That is why God is not ashamed to be called their God, for he has prepared a city for them. (Hebrews 11:13–16)

These were all men and women of great faith. It is stated that every one of them experienced the promise God gave him or her. For instance, in speaking of Joseph, it is stated in verse 22, "It was by faith that Joseph, when he was about to die, said confidently that the people of Israel would leave Egypt. He even commanded them to take his bones with them when they left." Joseph's faith allowed him to see something that would not actually happen for another 430 years. I find that astonishing. The children of Israel were kept in Egyptian slavery for 430 years waiting on deliverance from God. The fulfillment of God's promise to Joseph was 189 years longer than America has been a country. Please let that sink in. So often, we are so impatient when it comes to God's promises being fulfilled in our lives. Yet these great people of God, heroes of faith, never saw the promise fulfilled during their lifetimes. God on his part still greatly honored their faith.

All who have ever fought health issues want their miracle healings to occur immediately. As I've stated, that sometimes happens. It may occur more than I'll ever know. I hope and trust that's the case for you. I'm talking about miraculous healing here. That's when sickness and disease are corrected in a way only God could accomplish. Honest doctors and nurses will tell you about the many times they've seen things like this happen.

One Sunday morning, Pastor French interrupted his message and stated, "I feel the Lord is telling me that someone here has recently been diagnosed with cancer. If that person will come forward, we will pray for healing." Our hearts almost stopped. Corinne had just been informed the preceding Friday that she had cancer. We had called Pastor French that afternoon to inform him of that, but he was out of town. We decided to inform him of her diagnosis Sunday, but he was busy before the service, so we thought we would tell him after the service.

At the time, no one at church was aware of Corinne's situation. Then the surprise bomb was dropped. God gave Corinne a promise that morning; she believed she was healed, and a couple of months later, the healing was fully manifested. The time we waited for the manifestation was a time of great battle, but it ended in great victory. That took place over forty-one years ago, and she has never again had cancer.

On the other hand, I had to go through dramatic, invasive surgery to win my battle. I haven't spent too much time pondering that because I have been very secure in the peace God placed in me. However, the important thing here is that Corinne was healed and I wasn't, or at least not in the way we had expected me to be healed.

Shortly after my operation, Corinne asked God why I'd had had to have surgery to beat cancer but she hadn't. She felt the answer to her question was that she was still to be the mother of two more children. Prior to her cancer diagnosis, we had Scott, Chris, and Jule. We loved those kids and were very content with them. However, ten years later, Stacey was born, and in two more years, along came Ashley. We often tell people that we raised two families and have a laugh about that.

Corinne's miracle healing was much greater than the cancer being dispatched from her body; it included two more awesome people being born to this world. We not only experienced a miracle healing but two miracle babies as well! Once again, we must note that God's ways are not ours.

You may be wondering about the title of this chapter, "Everyone

Ignores These Bible Verses." I stated at the beginning of this chapter that probably more sermons have been given based on Hebrews 11 than any other chapter in the Bible. However, these sermons most likely have used verses 1–35a as the text and not verses 35b to the end of the chapter. For the sake of context, I'll quote these important verses as they fit into my thoughts regarding the subject of this book.

> But others were tortured, refusing to turn from God in order to be set free. They placed their hope in a better life after the resurrection. Some were jeered at, and their backs were cut open with whips. Others were chained in prison. Some died by stoning, some were sawed in half, and others were killed with the sword. Some went about wearing skins of sheep and goats, destitute and oppressed and mistreated. They were too good for this world, wandering over deserts and mountains, hiding in caves and holes in the ground. All these people earned a good reputation because of their faith, yet none of them received all that God had promised. For God had something better in mind for us, so that they would not reach perfection without us.

I've not heard many sermons preached based on these verses; no one wants to hear about suffering. But Paul or the writer of this letter wrote of people who were tortured, jeered at, whipped, chained, imprisoned, stoned to death, sawed in half, killed with swords, not clothed properly and "destitute and oppressed and mistreated." That certainly doesn't sound like the great life of health and prosperity TV preachers speak of. These people mentioned in this part of Hebrews didn't really enjoy the abundant life so many preachers promise us.

Sickness and disease aren't really mentioned in these verses. Rather, these people suffered in this life because of their faith in God. You might say that they were the martyrs of their day. However, we can connect sickness and disease with these afflictions as many of us who have had to deal with severe sickness and disease have also fought the battle of our lives. My entire body was not "sawed in half," but my neck sure was cut open end to end. I had asked God for a miracle, but the miracle I was seeking never came. I didn't know then that God had even greater things in store for me. Thankfully, I could rest in the fact that He was in control.

The Old Testament saints mentioned above were terribly afflicted. They, like you and I, sought God for deliverance. That deliverance never came; none of them received God's promise. Just think—they possibly trusted God for most of their lives while going through great afflictions believing God would soon deliver them from their affliction. But deliverance never came. Nonetheless, they continued to trust God and do what He asked them to do knowing something much greater was working on their behalf. At the time, they were unable to visualize God's full plan. Regardless, their walk with Him was such that they earned a good reputation because of their faith.

We too were brought into their situation and linked to them because the writer of Hebrews said in verse 40, "For God had something better in mind for us, so that they would not reach perfection without us." God's plan for them was far greater than their deliverance from their present afflictions. While their lives were memorials to their great faith, they would find their ultimate deliverance in the next life, where no persecution exists.

The great difference between these Old Testament Saints and us is Jesus Christ. They were alive before the cross, while we live after the cross and Christ's finished works. We live in the new covenant while they lived in the old covenant under the Law. When God looks at us, He sees His perfect plan for humanity in operation. When He sees us, He sees His Son. When God looks at me, He sees Christ in His Larry form. When He looks at you, He sees Christ in your form. When He looks at you, He does not see sickness, disease, failure, or even sin; He sees only Christ. In His Son and in you, He is well pleased!

My friend, please take comfort in God's words here. You may be going through a time of great and difficult trial. Your body may be riddled with pain. You have asked God to heal you, but He hasn't. Everything within you may be shouting out, "Why me, God? How much longer, God? I can't take it anymore!" I've seen that side of the coin. I pray right now that you too will join the millions who are experiencing miracle healing right this minute. Yet, if the miracle still seems to elude you, I pray you will see God's hand working in your life. I pray that you will be encouraged to remember He has absolute control of your life. Your faith in this fact tolerates no reason for you to be also suffering from fear, shame, or condemnation. God has not refused you healing because you are a second-class Christian. He isn't angry at you, nor is He punishing you because of the secret sin in your life.

God does not expect you to measure up to His higher standards by quoting and declaring more healing verses. No, He loves you because He can't do anything other than that! His divine healing miracle for you is not relegated by your works. And His plan for you just may go way beyond healing from sickness and disease. Again, His ways are not ours. I hope that you can begin to grasp this point.

In 1 Corinthians 12, Paul taught about the gifts of the Spirit. He also listed what are often called the ascension gifts—the apostles, prophets, teachers, those who performed miracles, those who had the gift of healing, those who helped others, those who had the gift of leadership, and those who spoke in unknown languages. Considering all the wonderful gifts Paul stated that God had given to the church, he ended this chapter with verse 31: "But now let me show you a way of life that is best of all." That, my friend, is what I wish to discuss next.

14

GOD'S ULTIMATE HEALING

Some may find this chapter upsetting. Others will take great comfort in it. I trust that you will find yourself in the latter group. We who have placed our faith and trust in God's plan for us through Jesus Christ should find comfort in the fact that we will always be in the presence of God.

As we live, we realize God's presence in us. He is as close as our next heartbeat. Christ in us is the core and heartbeat of the new-covenant grace message. We no longer find ourselves separated from God. It's impossible because we are His dwelling place, His new temple.

Look at Paul's words in Ephesians 2:19–22.

> So now you Gentiles are no longer strangers and foreigners. You are citizens along with all of God's holy people. You are members of God's family. Together, we are his house, built on the foundation of the apostles and prophets. And the cornerstone is Christ Jesus himself. We are carefully joined together in him, becoming a holy temple for the Lord. Through him you Gentiles are also being

made part of this dwelling where God lives by his
Spirit.

I find the concept of us being the holy temple for the Lord
breathtaking. While I live, no matter what condition I find myself
in—sickness or health, Christ lives in me and will never leave me.
Talk about comfort!

Yet this gets even better. I will be with my loving God for
eternity, and so will you. Paul told us in 1 Thessalonians 4:17, "Then
we will be with the Lord forever." Also, in that day, there will be no
sickness, disease, or even tears; those things will have ceased to exist.
John wrote in Revelation 21:3,

> I heard a loud shout from the throne, saying, "Look,
> God's home is now among his people! He will live
> with them, and they will be his people. God himself
> will be with them. He will wipe every tear from their
> eyes, and there will be no more death or sorrow or
> crying or pain. All these things are gone forever."

Keeping all this in mind, could death be God's ultimate healing?
If you have recently lost a loved one or a close friend, these words
may hit a tender spot in you. However, as we focus on the ongoing
relationship our loved ones or friends are now enjoying with God,
how can we do anything other than rejoice with them? There is no
way those who have passed from this life would ever wish to return.
I have made it very clear to my family and church, mostly in jesting,
but I'm very serious when I say, "When I die, no one is to pray me
back to life!" Please, when I'm in heaven, just leave me alone. I'll be
very upset with anyone who raises me from the dead.

The church has done a poor job teaching what heaven is all about.
As a result, the only time we hear of death is at memorial services.
We have failed to teach our people the rudiments of kingdom life.
Our mysterious writer of the book of Hebrews addressed some basic

kingdom doctrines that all believers should understand. Paul (Oops again! I mean the writer) said in Hebrews 6:1–3,

> So let us stop going over the basic teachings about Christ again and again. Let us go on instead and become mature in our understanding. Surely, we don't need to start again with the fundamental importance of repenting from evil deeds and placing our faith in God. You don't need further instruction about baptisms, the laying on of hands, the resurrection of the dead, and eternal judgment. And so, God willing, we will move forward to further understanding.

This writer stated that understanding the resurrection of the dead is a basic teaching of the church and that we should be going on from that into deeper truths. Yet many in the church today don't have even a basic understanding of heavenly things. The church is failing in this area and leaving its people without comfort when death touches their lives.

We can find comfort in the Bible on this subject.

> And now, dear brothers and sisters, we want you to know what will happen to the believers who have died so you will not grieve like people who have no hope. For since we believe that Jesus died and was raised to life again, we also believe that when Jesus returns, God will bring back with him the believers who have died. (1 Thessalonians 4:13–14)

> For the Lord himself will come down from heaven with a commanding shout, with the voice of the archangel, and with the trumpet call of God. First the Christians who have died will rise from their

graves. Then, together with them, we who are still alive and remain on the earth will be caught up in the clouds to meet the Lord in the air. So, encourage each other with these words. (1 Thessalonians 4:16–18)

For I fully expect and hope that I will never be ashamed, but that I will continue to be bold for Christ, as I have been in the past. And I trust that my life will bring honor to Christ, whether I live or die. For to me, living means living for Christ, and dying is even better. But if I live, I can do more fruitful work for Christ. So, I really don't know which is better. I'm torn between two desires: I long to go and be with Christ, which would be far better for me. But for your sakes, it is better that I continue to live. (Philippians 1:20–24)

That is why we never give up. Though our bodies are dying, our spirits are being renewed every day. (2 Corinthians 4:16)

Just as everyone dies because we all belong to Adam, everyone who belongs to Christ will be given new life. But there is an order to this resurrection: Christ was raised as the first of the harvest; then all who belong to Christ will be raised when he comes back. (1 Corinthians 15:22–23)

But let me reveal to you a wonderful secret. We will not all die, but we will all be transformed! It will happen in a moment, in the blink of an eye, when the last trumpet is blown. For when the trumpet sounds, those who have died will be raised to live forever. And we who are living will also be transformed. For our dying bodies must be transformed into bodies that will never die; our mortal bodies must be transformed into immortal bodies. Then when our dying bodies have been transformed into bodies that will never die, this scripture will be fulfilled: "Death is swallowed up in victory. O death, where is your victory? O death, where is your sting?" For sin is the sting that results in death, and the law gives sin its power. But thank God! He gives us victory over sin and death through our Lord Jesus Christ. So, my dear brothers and sisters, be strong and immovable. Always work enthusiastically for the Lord, for you know that nothing you do for the Lord is ever useless. (1 Corinthians 15:51–58)

I trust that these verses bless you nearly as much as they bless me. Paul made a powerful statement: "For our dying bodies must be transformed into bodies that will never die; our mortal bodies must be transformed into immortal bodies." It's impossible for flesh and blood to physically enter the kingdom of heaven. We live in the kingdom of God on earth, but one day, we will enter the kingdom of heaven and live there for eternity. To do that, we must die. I'm certain you've heard, "As soon as we were born, we began dying." This is a fact we will all face one day. We must have immortal bodies, and physical death is the only way this is possible. Death is nothing to fear. When we understand this, we will welcome it.

Is it good for a person to die before his or her time? No. For people to die before their time isn't good, but who can judge the timing? Only God. We look at a young person who died in an accident or due to sickness and say, "What a shame! He died so young, long before his time." Yet can we really say when our time to die is? Only God knows these things, and I rest in the knowledge that He has the plan for my life under control. Only God knows what problems a person is spared by experiencing death even at an early age.

Years ago, we pastored a church in the Midwest. Every spring and early summer, we would be hit with strong thunderstorms, many of which came with tornados. A woman in our church was deathly afraid of tornados. Whenever the sky would even hint that a storm was possible, she would hide in total fear.

I wondered about the worst thing a tornado could do to me; it could kill me. So, if I was in church worshiping the Lord and a huge twister fell from the sky and killed me right on the spot, the next second I'd be in the eternal, physical presence of God. How could that be a fearful, dreaded thing?

Prior to my surgery, the cancer began to spread rapidly. I could see the concern on my two oncologists' faces. They had observed this many times and knew that if something—the chemo or the radiation—didn't work soon, most likely I'd die and soon. Later, when I was informed about the risks of the surgery, I was again exposed to my immortality. The cancer might kill me, or the surgery might do me in. Either way, things didn't look positive. However, my attitude was the same as it was about those Midwest tornados. What's the worst that could happen? If I didn't survive the cancer or the operation, oh well. I'd just awaken in the eternal presence of the Lord. There was nothing to fear in this win/win situation.

The most difficult aspect of death is the effect it has on loving survivors. My dad has been gone for quite a few years now. The other day was Memorial Day. To celebrate the day and my dad's life, I posted an old picture of him in his navy uniform on my Facebook page. He served on a battleship during World War II. That same picture of dad is my current screen saver on my cell phone, and I see that picture several times a day. Yet when I posted the picture on Facebook, tears came to my eyes. I'll never forget my dad; memories of him will always bring tears to my eyes. I miss him, but there's no way I'd ever wish him to come back to this life. He is so much better off now!

I mentioned before the possibly this chapter might hit a tender spot in you. Maybe you have recently lost a loved one to death and reading these words is creating uncomfortable emotions. If that's the case, remember the healing effect of time. Every day of your life, your mourning will become less disturbing. Once again, the one-day-at-a-time approach works wonders; your emotions will heal.

If you've received a death-sentence prediction due to a current condition in your body, realize you have nothing to fear. Years ago, I sensed that the Holy Spirit gave me some revelation on death. I felt that death could be compared to stepping over a small stream. As a young man living in Michigan, I was brought up on trout fishing. Many excellent trout streams and rivers were within an hour's drive. However, all over the area were little brooks meandering through woods and cow pastures. The current would undercut a bank here or there leaving a shady hole maybe two feet deep. Hiding in that hole would be a nice brook trout just waiting for my hook covered with a bit of worm to drift through that hole. These trout would be less than a foot long; catching one seven inches long, the legal limit those days, was a real feat. The reward of a creel full of these fish was the best, sweetest fish dinner one could ever have.

These little brooks could easily be crossed over with a single step. That's how I eventually saw death. On one side of the brook was temporal life, and on the other side was life eternal. It was just a very simple crossover. Just as there was never any effort involved in crossing one of those narrow brooks, there is never any effort involved in crossing over into eternal life. However, the significant blessing is that as we cross over the brook of death, we end up eternally in the arms of God. This is not a sad thing at all.

In writing about the new bodies that believers in Christ would one day have after death, Paul shared many thoughts with the church in Corinth. Please take comfort from his words in 2 Corinthians 5:1–8.

For we know that when this earthly tent we live in is taken down (that is, when we die and leave this earthly body), we will have a house in heaven, an eternal body made for us by God himself and not by human hands. We grow weary in our present bodies, and we long to put on our heavenly bodies like new clothing. For we will put on heavenly bodies; we will not be spirits without bodies. While we live in these earthly bodies, we groan and sigh, but it's not that we want to die and get rid of these bodies that clothe us. Rather, we want to put on our new bodies so that these dying bodies will be swallowed up by life. God himself has prepared us for this, and as a guarantee he has given us his Holy Spirit.

So, we are always confident, even though we know that as long as we live in these bodies we are not at home with the Lord. For we live by believing and not by seeing. Yes, we are fully confident, and we would rather be away from these earthly bodies, for then we will be at home with the Lord.

Yes, our earthly bodies are dying. That process began the minute we were born. We will all die, and sickness and disease can be an unwelcome part of the process. However, in this life, we are preparing for the next life, where death, sickness, and disease no longer exist. I trust you too are looking forward to that day. We can't lose. If we are miraculously healed or slowly recover from illness in this life, we win. On the other hand, if we cross that brook, we win as well—we receive the ultimate prize.

Final Thoughts

I hope this book has been a blessing to you. It's been a tremendous blessing to me because writing about my bout with cancer has helped bring more emotional healing to my life. My battle took a toll on me, one I'm slowly rebounding from. My thoughts about God's healing process have been completely transformed and reinforced by writing this book. For me, this has been a good thing.

I didn't want to write an exhaustive, deep, theological position paper on the doctrines of divine healing. Often in writing, I had to purposely avoid the temptation of getting into the weeds. The people in my church know how easily I can get sidetracked in my teaching. I think I've done a pretty good job of avoiding the bunny trails. At least I hope so. I wanted to communicate my journey through the dark days of cancer, surgery, and the long recovery and present my thoughts on God's love and healing, which I hope will help and bless my readers.

I would like to revisit the main title of this work, *When God Doesn't Heal*. I trust that after reading my thoughts, you see that my title is more of an attention getter than a theological statement because God always heals! However, His healing may not come in the way we expect. I hope I've made this point very clear.

Second, in no way do I wish to discourage anyone from trusting God for a physical healing miracle. God moves in diverse ways in different people; no one way is the right way for everyone. I have a very close friend who's going through some grave physical conditions.

He is committed to believing God for his miracle healing; he has chosen not to pursue medical treatment other than occasional doctor checkups. My friend needs a miracle to save his life. I support him in his stand. However, even if he chose to seek medical treatment, I'd still totally support him. He can hear from God in his situation, and his decision is completely the proper path for him to take no matter what I think.

If you are seeking God for a physical healing from some sort of sickness or disease, I encourage you to keep seeking it. However, if in your seeking you somehow have fallen into the trap of legalistic thinking on the subject, I encourage you to look at the proper balance on the matter. If you have ultimately fallen into some form of fear, shame, or condemnation, I trust you can recognize this and reject whatever it was that brought you to that place. If by reading this book you can do the above, I will consider this book a significant success.

I'm currently eight months and twelve days post-surgery. A recent CT scan showed no ongoing cancer in my head or neck. For me to be considered officially cancer free, I must remain clean for five years. A week ago, I celebrated my seventieth birthday. It's amazing what facing death can do to your understanding of and appreciation for life. I feel I'll never have to face cancer again; I'll breeze right past that five-year mark.

The physical condition of my face and neck is improving. My neck is somewhat deformed due to the removal of my lymph nodes, so I must at times deal with some swelling. My mouth is improving. The flap, the new tissue, is becoming a normal part of life. I often have difficulty moving food around it, so food frequently gets stuck behind it. My tongue was also intensely affected. I no longer can lick a postage stamp; I must get my finger wet to do that. And I still don't have any lower teeth. Folks at the University of Florida's dental clinic told me it would be best to wait until I'm two years post-surgery before even considering dental implants.

A recent development is that a very small section, smaller than a pinkie fingertip, of my new jawbone has broken through the skin in the right gum line. Due to this, the right side of my tongue is becoming irritated when I speak. There isn't much that can be done about that. We were hoping that new skin would form over the exposed bone. Two bone fragments were eventually pulled out of my gum line, and that gave me immediate relief. I can eat most things, including tender meat. Just last evening, we had a Family Fun Night at our church. We enjoyed catered fried chicken and pulled pork. I could easily eat the pork; however, the chicken was a little dry, so I had a challenging time eating that.

I still don't have any feeling in my lower chin, jaw, and upper neck, so I continue to make a mess while eating. I go through a pile of napkins at every meal because I can't feel any food running down my chin.

But I can talk. That's a miracle! I preach most Sunday mornings these days, and people tell me they can understand what I say. Sometimes, I have a tough time understanding myself. I must work at speaking. Usually, I try to avoid small talk. Most people take speaking for granted. However, I must work at enunciation. After speaking a lot, I often end up tired. I trust that I'm learning how to become an effective communicator though I'm a man of fewer spoken words now.

My right leg is healed. I have a huge scar on the right side, where the bone that became my new jawbone was removed. That's also where tissue was removed to become the flap in my mouth. I enjoy telling people that that's where I was bitten by a gator—a Florida joke.

Above my right knee, I have two red patches about eight inches long and two inches wide. These patches are where the skin grafts were taken to put on my lower leg. They're healing very well, and normal color is slowly returning to the skin.

I have also lost a lot of weight through this process, nearly a hundred pounds. Losing the weight was great, but the way it was done wasn't so wonderful. In the early days of treatment, the doctors kept telling me to not lose weight. I used to laugh at that because all my life, doctors had told me to lose weight!

Overall, I'm doing very well. I most likely will never return to the ways things used to be. I may talk funny for the rest of my life. However, I can talk, and I'm alive. All I can say to that is "Glory!" However, as of today, September 15, 2017, the 1st Year Anniversary of my surgery, I have been confronted with a new development. A couple of weeks ago, during a routine appointment with Dr. Boyce, he suspected a problem with a lymph node on the lower right side of my neck. He ordered a CT scan, which showed results of "recurrent metastatic confluent nodal mass centered in the right level 4 region." In layman's terms, it simply means that there is the possibility that a lymph node is cancerous. In doing some research of my own, I've discovered that this is a very common situation with patients who have gone through what I've gone through. The immediate follow-up is a scheduled biopsy to be done this coming Monday morning. I then have another appointment with Dr. Boyce to discuss further treatment. So, you see, my battle is ongoing! However, I do feel good. I have complete peace about all of this and I am assured that everything that I've written in this book still stands. God knows my situation. I rest in that! Unfortunately, you my Reader, will not know the future outcome of my life. However, if you follow me on Social Media or know me in any other way, you will know.

If you ever think to pray for me, I certainly would appreciate it; I would count it an honor. I feel that by reading my book, you too have become one of my guardian angels and thus an integral part of my support team. Though I may not know you, I trust I have become a part of your support team as well!

Therefore, here is my prayer for you.

Father, in the name of Jesus, I pray for those reading my book. Most likely, they have read this book because they are in some way involved in dealing with sickness or disease, maybe even a life-or-death situation. We acknowledge You as our healer. We know that Your ways are much higher than ours. Therefore, You have the perfect path of healing already planned for them. I thank You for this plan.

I also speak life and health to my readers. I command all sickness and disease to die in them and pass harmlessly from them. I thank You for healing them in any way You choose. Your love for them will never leave. If they are facing any fear, shame, and condemnation, I pray that too will be removed from their lives and thus allow them to come into the full revelations of Your new-covenant love, completely transforming their lives.

Father, I thank You for them. In the name of Jesus, I pray, amen.

May God our Father and the Lord Jesus Christ give you grace and peace.

Printed in the United States
By Bookmasters